Probation Round the World

While they retain a recognizable common core, probation systems around the world are enormously varied and many are in a state of rapid change. *Probation Round the World* is a study of probation in ten countries, ranging from the well-resourced and heavily professionalized services of Britain and the old Commonwealth to the reliance on lay-supervisors in Japan and the community-based system which has recently been set up in Papua New Guinea.

Probation Round the World is the result of collaborative research involving the United Nations Interregional Crime and Justice Research Institute (UNICRI), the British Home Office and experts in the ten countries in the study: Australia, Canada, Hungary, Israel, Japan, Papua New Guinea, the Philippines, Sweden, England and Wales, and Scotland. The results paint a picture of probation systems in a state of flux. Faced with rising crime, the more industrialized countries have placed renewed importance on probation as a means not only of reducing reoffending, but also of containing burgeoning prison populations. This has led to more overtly 'correctionalist' systems than before, as probation clienteles include a growing proportion of more serious offenders.

Theoretically innovative, *Probation Round the World* assesses the state of comparative research on probation and offers a coherent and in-depth analysis of probation in the ten countries in the study.

Koichi Hamai is an International Liaison Officer at the International Affairs Office, Corrections Bureau, Ministry of Justice, Japan; **Robert Harris** is Professor of Social Work at the University of Hull; **Mike Hough** is Professor of Social Policy at South Bank University, London; **Renaud Villé** is an Associate Research Officer and **Ugljesa Zvekic** is Research Co-ordinator, both at UNICRI in Rome.

Probation Round the World

A comparative study

Edited by Koichi Hamai,
Renaud Villé, Robert Harris,
Mike Hough and Ugljesa Zvekic

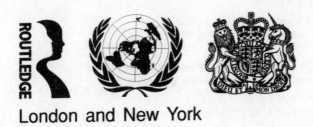

London and New York

First published 1995 by Routledge
11 New Fetter Lane, London EC4P 4EE

Simultaneously published in the USA and Canada
by Routledge, 29 West 35th Street, New York, NY 10001

© 1995 UNICRI, British Home Office and Robert Harris

Typeset in Times Ten 10/12 by
Florencetype Ltd, Stoodleigh, Devon

Printed and bound in Great Britain by
Clays Ltd, St Ives plc

British Library Cataloguing in Publication Data
A catalogue record for this book is available from
the British Library

Library of Congress Cataloguing in Publication Data
A catalogue record for this book has been requested

ISBN   0-415-11516-7 (hbk)
ISBN   0-415-11517-5 (pbk)

Contents

Illustrations

BOXES

Preface

Whilst there is a worldwide search for credible new non-custodial sanctions, some traditional ones such as probation have received insufficient attention from comparative research. True, as this book shows, high quality work has been carried out and is still underway in, for example, Europe and Asia. Yet, attempts towards wider 'comparative imagination' in this area were almost non-existent for several decades. This is somewhat surprising in view both of the number of countries introducing probation and of developments and reforms in those systems with probation as a tradition.

The Research Workshop on Alternatives to Imprisonment organized by the United Nations Interregional Crime and Justice Research Institute (UNICRI) at the Eighth United Nations Congress on the Prevention of Crime and the Treatment of Offenders (Havana, Cuba, 1990) noted this neglect and recommended, among other things, a greater use of and research into traditional non-custodial sanctions, including probation.

If this provided the initial impetus for the project reported here, our two institutions seemed particularly well placed to collaborate on it. The origins of probation can be traced to the British legal system, and a substantial record of probation research made the Home Office Research and Statistics Department an appropriate contributor. On the other hand, UNICRI's continuous involvement in international comparative research in crime and criminal justice, and as mentioned above, more recently in the area of non-custodial sanctions, made this an especially appropriate partnership, the results of which we are most pleased to present here.

Our thanks go to the contributing experts and to the editors of this volume as well as to Routledge for the interest shown in our work.

Christopher Nuttall
Director
Research and Statistics Department,
Home Office,
London

Herman F. Woltring
Director
United Nations Interregional
Crime and Justice Research Institute,
Rome

October 1994

Acknowledgements

The debts which accrue in any research are usually considerable; they are the more so in cross-national studies, where the researchers depend on colleagues with whom face-to-face contact is necessarily limited. Thanks are due in particular to the local experts, who with generosity, enthusiasm and commitment gave of their expertise, and without whom the book could not have been written. They are as follows:

Australia	1 Mr Robert Fitzgerald, Executive Director, Strategic and Specialist Services, Ministry of Justice, Western Australia
	2 Mr Brad Miles, Programme Development Officer, New South Wales Probation Service
	3 Mr Peter Visser, Co-ordinator, Community Corrections Development, Department of Correctional Services, South Australia
Canada	Mr Gordon Parry, Co-ordinator, Sentencing Team, Department of Justice
England and Wales	Mr Mike Hough, formerly Senior Principal Research Officer, Research and Planning Unit, Home Office; now Professor, South Bank University, London
Hungary	1 Judge Piroska Versitz, Dunakeszi District Court
	2 Mr Károly Horváth, Probation Officer and Secretary of the National Association of Probation Officers

Israel	Mr Meir Hovav, Director, Division of Youth Development and Correctional Services, Ministry of Labour and Social Affairs
Japan	Professor Takashi Kubo, Research and Training Institute, Ministry of Justice
Papua New Guinea	Mr Leo Tohichem, Chief Probation Officer, Probation and Parole and Juvenile Courts Services, Department of Attorney-General
The Philippines	Mr Francisco Ruivivar, Administrator, Parole and Probation Administration, Department of Justice
Scotland	Mr Felim O'Leary, Assistant Chief Inspector, Social Work Services Inspectorate, Social Work Services Group, Scottish Home and Health Department
Sweden	Ms Ann Sandberg, Senior Administrative Officer, Division for Treatment and Production, Swedish Prison and Probation Administration

We are grateful too for help offered in the course of this study by Professor Menachim Amir (Israel), Dr David Biles (Australia), Dr Frederick Greenwald (USA), Mr Harri Montonen (Finland), Professor Herschel Prins (England), Ms Mirjana Tomic-Malic (Netherlands) and Miss Alison Wakefield (England).

We acknowledge our indebtedness to our employing institutions, the Home Office (in particular Mr Christopher Nuttall, Director of Research and Statistics), UNICRI and the University of Hull; and to the University of Cambridge Institute of Criminology for library assistance. Particular thanks for unflagging secretarial support are due to Anne Baroni (UNICRI), Jean Bartlett (Home Office) and Jane Rymer (University of Hull).

Editors' introduction

*Koichi Hamai, Renaud Villé, Robert Harris,
Mike Hough and Ugljesa Zvekic*

... probation belongs to those subjects which call for an international exchange of new ideas and actual experience. The
forms of legal institutions must be so designed that they fit into
the framework of the national system of law, but treatment
implies a personal relationship and thus is a general human
problem that knows no frontier and has long been the subject
of human co-operation.

(United Nations 1954a: 2–3)

Probation has for a long time been an aspect of many criminal
justice systems. This book is the first study of probation round
the world outside a purely regional context, and it offers a
conceptual as well as descriptive account of how different
probation systems operate. It aims to address the needs of policy
makers, theoreticians, researchers and practitioners of probation
and criminal justice in both the developed and the developing
worlds.

For readers in the developed world our aim is to set the themes
and issues which dominate professional assumptions and activities
in a broader context. This is intended not only to be informative
and interesting in itself but to invite the development of what
we might term a *comparative imagination*. Developing such an
imagination necessitates a willingness to regard oneself as a partic-
ipant in a complex and variegated international enterprise. This
in turn involves decentring one's professional preoccupations
by locating them in a larger and more diverse context. Hence
we must suspend temporarily our preoccupation with the exigen-
cies of the moment and embrace, cognitively and affectively, the
notion that the activities of our counterparts in, for example,

Sweden, Australia or the Philippines fall within our proper professional domain, enabling us to see our parochial concerns from different legal and cultural perspectives. Hence, in a comparative context:

> the purpose of cultural comparison should be to contribute to internal debate and development by providing an abrasive challenge to the routine assumption framework within which that debate and development tend to occur. Rather than allowing superficial appearances to disguise the conceptually unfamiliar, comparative analysis which provokes conceptual challenge may enhance the development of a distinctive probation culture.
>
> (Clear and Rumgay 1992: 10)

A comparative imagination takes us beyond both the discredited notion that unilaterally exporting knowledge from the developed to the developing world is desirable and the seemingly progressive but in practice often patronizing courtesy that 'we' in the developed world have much to learn from developing nations. While the principle is precisely correct, for we do indeed have much to learn, the evidence of such learning having taken place is somewhat sparse, and it is hard to avoid the conclusion that in some spheres of human activity at least we know too little either of what there is to learn or how to learn it.

To deal with this problem of cross-national learning by simply trying to convert the imperialist belief in the unilateral export of law and administration into a bilateral process whereby developed nations voluntarily receive from the developing nations what was once imposed on them may be an advance, but only a limited one. Indeed, if anything, it legitimates the idea that such learning can be based on administrative emulation or cultural transportation. While the possibility of picking up good ideas from overseas is by no means to be decried – and in this book we discuss a number of practices worthy of consideration elsewhere – it would be too narrow to take the possibility of picking up handy hints from foreigners as sufficient justification for cross-national study.

The learning to be had is above all about oneself and one's assumptive world, and about the artificial boundaries on professional development imposed by those forms of nation-state thinking which discourage the exercise of a comparative imagination. And examples of nation-state thinking abound: too often overseas study visits are thought of as a paid holiday and not funded; too often they are not fully reported on or evaluated on completion; too often the probation officer in Birmingham Alabama or Birmingham England regards the work of the probation service in Papua New Guinea or Sweden as 'outside of' his or her professional ambit because it is 'different'. The comparative imagination on the other hand, faced with the complaint that because probation overseas is 'different' it is therefore 'irrelevant', responds that on the contrary it is this very difference which makes such activities pressingly relevant.

While, therefore, this book contains useful thoughts and possibilities for developed world readers and much that is worthy of discussion, for these possibilities to be realized certain demands are made of readers too. Above all, the book needs to be read in a spirit of genuine interest and enquiry, not as a scavenger aiming to exploit someone else's work for domestic purposes. For to take such an approach is actually to narrow one's vision so, paradoxically, reducing the yield of helpful ideas available for assimilation.

Not surprisingly, we hope readers in the developing world will include those considering the introduction of probation into their own criminal justice systems. It follows from what has been said, however, that for them we aim to be constructive but not prescriptive. In particular, we hope, by explaining and discussing the range of probation models throughout the world, to discourage the unthinking imitation of North American, Australian, or English/ Welsh models which, while they may work in those countries, may be undesirable or unnecessary in the developing world. After all, though the legacy of professional imperialism has by no means been uniformly malevolent (Igbinovia 1989) it has certainly had well-documented negative consequences (Clifford 1974; Midgley 1977; Brillon 1980; Cohen 1982; Mandal 1989; Rotimi and Oloruntimehin 1992) and we should not wish them to be increased as a result of our work. One Indian writer, for example, noting that in the post-war period some 90 per cent of books in a government bibliography on social welfare in India were imported, notes that:

Even today, there is no basic textbook on Indian social work which takes into consideration indigenous elements of social,

economic and political life. India has found a ready-made body
of formulated concepts, principles, theories and techniques in
US social work.

(Nagpaul 1993: 211)

On the other hand, we certainly do not wish to discourage
sensible appropriation: traditional modes of justice should not be
idealized, for many of them include practices which are viewed
by the international community as ineffective if not abhorrent and
few, unchanged, will have the capacity to meet the challenges
which countries in the developing world currently face. For any
country struggling to develop new penalties in a criminal justice
system based on incarceration, mutilation or revenge, the value
of conditionality, the demands made on the offender, the penalties imposed for not meeting these demands, the nature of the
relationship between the offender and the supervisor, the training
of the supervisor or the involvement of traditional support or
control networks require local discussion and resolution. We hope,
however, that such discussions and solutions may be informed by
the experience of those with knowledge of making probation
systems work and that this book will contribute to the quality of
this debate.

The field of comparative probation has been surprisingly under-
investigated. For example, there nowhere exists a census of
probation systems throughout the world, nor is there any study
of whether or how countries without a probation service provide
information to courts or supervise offenders. There has been
no comparative study of probation in developing countries –
how it relates to traditional forms of justice, how it secures
community support, whether it uses members of the community
as volunteers. In fact, there has been no recent study of whether
there is in fact any such 'thing' as probation in an international
context, or whether people called 'probation officers' are united
in name only and perform quite different functions in different
countries.

Within the framework of the United Nations crime prevention
and criminal justice programme, this study represents a follow-
up to the UNICRI-organized Research Workshop on Alternatives
to Imprisonment held at the Eighth United Nations Congress on
the Prevention of Crime and the Treatment of Offenders (Havana,
Cuba, 27 August – 7 September 1990). The Workshop paid special

attention to the factors promoting the use of non-custodial sanctions and noted, *inter alia*, that:

> the most efficient route to increase the credibility of non-custodial sanctions and thus promote their use is for the state and local community to provide the necessary resources and financial support for the development, enforcement and monitoring of such sanctions. Particular attention should also be paid to the training of the practitioners responsible for the implementation of the sanctions and for co-ordination between criminal justice agencies and other agencies involved in the implementation of these sanctions in the community.
>
> (Zvekic 1994: 23)

The Congress also adopted the resolution on principles and directions for research on non-custodial sanctions. The resolution in particular highlighted the need to promote

> research on the use and effectiveness of non-custodial sanctions in order to facilitate the making of informed decisions.
>
> (United Nations 1990: 155)

It is then within this framework that the UNICRI and the Home Office reached an agreement to carry out this study, the results of which are presented in this volume.

THE PRESENT STUDY

The core of the project was an empirical study of a variety of different probation systems. The study focused on eleven systems in nine countries and one well-documented and interesting country which lacks such a system, Scotland, where different arrangements apply for the set of tasks normally undertaken by probation officers. Using these case studies – which cover three states in Australia, Canada, England and Wales, Hungary, Israel, Japan, Papua New Guinea, the Philippines, Scotland and Sweden – we have provided accounts of the operation of each system, and have aimed to identify both common (or defining) features and significant variations.

Our aim in producing the book has been to provide some reliable comparative material not only on the uses and benefits of probation, but also on problems faced by criminal justice systems in operating probation systems effectively.

International Bibliography on Probation

At the start of the study, we prepared an International Bibliography on Probation,[1] to identify the issues, previous research and the countries which have probation services. The Bibliography comprises about 1,700 titles (books and articles) and refers to research carried out from 1980 up until 1992. Most of the references were located from material held by the UNICRI Documentation Centre or from major international abstract journals. Keywords have been also identified and attached to the entries.

Definition of probation

The next step was to define what we meant by probation. Although the concept of probation has wide currency, there is no clear definition of probation in different criminal justice systems. We defined a system as a probation system if it satisfied the following criteria:

- *Distinct organization*: the administration of the probation system should be dealt with separately within the criminal justice system;

- *Judicial function*: probation should have a judicial function in the criminal justice system and placing a person on probation should be the result of a judicial decision;

- *Legal mandate*: probation should be based on a legal mandate;

- *Supervision*: being placed on probation should imply that the offender receives supervision (in this study, the conditional release of an offender, without supervision, is not considered probation);

- *In the community*: probation should not only control offenders but it should also help them to readjust in the community.

Our research has focused more on conventional probation for adults, and has covered only in passing related areas such as parole, community service orders and restitution. We have focused on probation as opposed to parole in view of the UN interest in promoting probation as an alternative to imprisonment.

Identification of the countries

On the basis of previous studies and personal contacts, we prepared a fairly comprehensive chart of probation systems in different countries. We selected systems from the chart which (a) met our criteria and (b) gave a broad geographical spread. The study did not include countries where probation exists only in vestigial form – for example where legislation has provided for probation, but systems have not yet been firmly established. A state in a country with a federal system, such as Australia, is regarded as a distinct unit due to differences in criminal justice systems and policies. While probation services in Canada are organized by provincial governments, those are operated under the same laws. Therefore, even though Canada is composed of different provinces, we have generally treated Canada as one unit.

Identification of experts

After identifying the countries, the next step was to identify national experts from each country. The identified countries were asked to provide us with a list of candidates. The national experts had to meet the following criteria:

- professional career in the probation service or relevant experience in research and evaluation of the probation system;

- a good command of the English language.

Drafting the questionnaire

Once selected, the experts were requested to complete a questionnaire. This was carefully drafted to avoid a culturally biased framework, and it contained both closed and open-ended questions. To give the experts an indication of the sort of depth and coverage we wanted, the draft national report from England and Wales was prepared in advance and was circulated as a template.

Expert Meeting

An Expert Meeting was organized to discuss the draft national reports, and to clarify the problems or difficulties that the experts may have had in completing the questionnaire (only the Canadian and Australian experts were unable to attend). Detailed discussions took place to ensure the questions were understood and appropriately answered, and arrangements were made to ensure that the study itself, and its main output, this book, were subject to careful checking and cross-checking. An individual interview with each national expert was organized in order to clarify some aspects of the draft national report, mainly those which are specific to the country. It was clearly important that the conclusions in particular were based upon a correct understanding of the individual responses.

Editorial board

The functioning of the Editorial Board is perhaps of interest given the nature and content of the study. The Board met on some six occasions in the course of a series of two-day sessions in Rome and London. Though the Board operated throughout as a team it divided tasks equitably among its members, with the Board as a whole taking responsibility for the final product. Ugljesa Zvekic took substantial responsibility for overall co-ordination of the project and in particular for liaison with local experts, supervision and overseeing Part II; Koichi Hamai and Renaud Villé designed the questionnaire, prepared all the tables and figures and were responsible for collating and first editing of materials from the local experts and redrafting; Mike Hough, who acted as England and Wales expert, was responsible for Chapter 7 and took responsibility for final editing of the rest of Part II; and Robert Harris was responsible for Chapters 1, 2 and 9.

STRUCTURE OF THE BOOK

The book comprises two parts. Part I discusses the nature of comparative research and provides an overview of origins, historical trends and development of probation. Part II presents material from the comparative case studies, and ends with a comparative analysis of the case studies.

Most of the information included in Part II has been extracted from the national reports which were prepared by the national experts in each of the participating countries. Some of the material has simply been reproduced or précised. Elsewhere we have summarized the information in the form of tables and figures; and when appropriate we have synthesized the material to draw out what struck us as the key points of similarity and difference between the systems.

It is our hope that this volume will contribute to the advance of international comparative research and to the appropriate diffusion of experience among different probation systems around the world. It will, we hope, also contribute to further co-operation between policy and research, and to an appreciation of the value of probation.

NOTES

1 The working draft of the International Bibliography on Probation is available from UNICRI (Via Giulia 52, 00186 Rome, Italy, Tel: +39/6/6877437, Fax: +39/6/6892638) on diskette upon request for US$ 10.

Part I

Comparative probation: some theoretical, methodological and empirical considerations

Chapter 1

Studying probation
A comparative approach

Robert Harris

> The particular importance of comparative social research is
> that it permits the discovery of possible universals, the specifi-
> cation of which empirical regularities are system-specific, the
> reassignment of rules not only as intrasystemic or extrasystemic
> but within those categories ... and, finally, the reexamination
> of concepts and methodologies that is mandated by the
> discovery of exceptions.
>
> (Grimshaw 1973: 15)

Comparative researchers face a number of potential pitfalls and
this is as much the case for researchers in the field of probation
as for others. Certainly any *a priori* assumption that probation is
a readily identifiable 'thing' replicable with only administrative
variation in different criminal justice systems should be viewed
with scepticism: probation itself requires first problematizing and
then clarifying. It does not, however, follow that a relativism which
decrees that 'anything' can constitute probation must ensue. After
all, probation round the world must presumably possess certain
characteristics for it to be rendered recognizable, even if what
those characteristics are is contested.

One quite precise definition of probation has been offered but
perhaps fails to encapsulate the range of systems across the world,
as opposed to those in the developed world:

> Probation is a method of punishment with a socio-pedagogic
> basis, characterised by a combination of supervision and assis-
> tance. It is applied under the free system to offenders selected
> according to their criminological personality and their recep-
> tiveness, in relation to a system whose aim is to give the subject
> the chance of modifying his approach to life in society and

to take his place in the social environment of his choice without the risk of violating a penal norm again.

(Cartledge *et al.* 1981: 22)

Our starting point is an earlier, less precise definition offered by the United Nations almost half a century ago which contains assumptions recognizable in almost all probation jurisdictions today:

probation is a method of dealing with specially selected offenders and ... consists of the conditional suspension of punishment while the offender is placed under personal supervision and is given individual guidance or 'treatment'.

(United Nations 1951: 4)

This definition contains four main elements: offenders must be *selected* as suitable; a *conditional suspension of punishment* is entailed; there is an element of *personal supervision*; and this involves *guidance or treatment*. With the caveat that, as will become clear, the conflation of probation and supervision has not been historically invariable and that 'conditional suspension of punishment' will emerge as more complicated than it may seem, we say something about each in turn.

SELECTION

The dimension of *selection* does not of itself take us far, for other than in respect of mandatory sentences a process of selection must precede any determination. With probation, however, when the UN definition is set in the context of the document as a whole it implies a particular character of and procedure for selection, hinted at in the use of the adverb 'specially'. This is the more so when we recall that the title of a key UN publication was *The Selection of Offenders for Probation* (United Nations 1959).

If, too, we read 'specially' correctly, as involving individual rather than category selection (as might operate in the routine application of a small fine for minor theft), the selection is likely to have been made on grounds tangential to legal variables surrounding the offence (such as gravity, intent or prior criminal record) but central to the perceived psychopathology, or at least personal characteristics of the offender. This implies a mode of selection in which the influence of the human or social science expert strongly influences the decision of the legal expert. Hence the document notes also:

> Probation is an essentially modern method for the treatment of offenders and as such, it is rooted in the broader social and cultural trends of the modern era ... This modern trend coincides with attempts to prevent crime by the improvement of social conditions and by development of social services. It is characterized, furthermore, by the recognition of the social rehabilitation of the individual offender as a main object of penal policy, and by the rational selection and development of effective means to this end.
>
> (United Nations 1951: 15)

And again:

> the considerations specified as those to which the court should have regard in selecting offenders for release on probation, should not only be compatible with, but should be directly related to, the essential purpose of probation. ... The only appropriate criteria seem to be (a) the amenability of a specific offender to successful treatment on probation, and (b) the consideration of general prevention.
>
> (United Nations 1951: 231)

The centrality of the experts in determinations is not, however, constitutive of probation, and a willingness to revere probation officers as powerful therapists is no prerequisite for the establishment of a probation system. Indeed, as the years up to 1951 saw in many countries the gradual displacement of the legal by the therapeutic discourse in relation to probation, so have the years since 1951 seen a move away from the therapeutic principles of the UN document in the majority of developed probation systems, not back to a principle of unsullied legalism but towards increasing juridical control of the experts.

It would be too simple to perceive this reversion to justice merely as a crude response to a more punitive environment: though it is true that such an environment exists in a number of western nations, the toughening of punishment is as much product as cause of the various political and economic transformations which have taken place. These transformations include:

- *The deteriorating world economic situation* following the oil crisis of the mid-1970s. Economic recession is characteristically detrimental to liberal social policies, and in particular there is evidence of an association between such recession and a reversion to the principles of classical justice (Paternoster and Bynum 1982).

- *The empirical limitations of therapeutic endeavours* which have come to be exposed by the increasing attention now paid to the relative effectiveness of different professional tactics. The conventional position today is more optimistic than that of the 1970s when a mood of nihilism, usually referred to in shorthand as 'nothing works', based on what was arguably a misreading of an influential 'evaluation of evaluations' (Martinson 1974), was *à la mode*. Nevertheless, even if we accept that some things sometimes work, evaluation research has too often fallen back on a methodology more suited to clinical drug trials than the evaluation of the intricate work of individual professionals working with individual offenders. In particular, by comparing different therapies and regarding professionals as interchangeable variables – taking supervision as a constant irrespective of the individual inputs of officer and offender – much evaluation research presents a model of probation as amenable to randomized application. Beyond this, however, little credence is currently accorded theories which, by granting aetiological status to individual psychopathology, justify a social response based on clinical treatment. Accordingly a return to the relatively unbridled power of the expert is almost nowhere a plausible political reality.

- In a number of major western countries since the 1970s the *therapeutic professions have come under pressure* not only from the new right but from the radical left, who have regarded their extensive therapeutic powers as covert social control (Cohen 1985). This pincer movement has if anything strengthened during the 1980s and early 1990s. From the right's specific attack on social professionals for tending, in Mrs Thatcher's phrase, to produce 'sociological alibis' for bad acts has emerged a broader-based critique of the role and function of professionals generally. Hence, in the United Kingdom, the 1980s have seen:

> the removal of professional monopolies (such as those of solicitors and opticians), funding squeezes and job losses (for

example in the Universities). Similarly, the decade has witnessed a transformation of the employment conditions of doctors and other health workers, the introduction of a national curriculum in schools, and radical proposals for the reform of our antiquated but powerful legal system. Scrutiny units have been instituted, with independent private sector expertise bought-in, and civil servants in particular have been subjected to hitherto unimagined forms of monitoring. New auditing agencies have been formed and existing regulatory institutions given enhanced authority. In short, the élites have felt a similar cold draught to that which has traditionally chilled mainly blue collar workers.

(Harris 1994: 38–9)

The challenge from the left has diversified too, from a predominantly class-based platform during the 1970s and early 1980s which perceived professional action as imposing middle-class norms on working-class families (see for example Donzelot 1980; Meyer 1983; Harris and Timms 1993a) to a more specific critique that to give undue discretion to individuals is to give free rein to systematic discrimination against already disadvantaged social groups (see for example Hudson 1993). This perspective has coalesced perfectly with the concern of the right to 'manage' professionals to justify the formation of an increasingly 'evaluative state' (Henkel 1991a; 1991b).

Though the UN document of 1951 presupposes that selection is based on therapeutic criteria, subsequent events have seen probation become increasingly central in penal policy in the west at a time when psychopathology has been widely repudiated as a general cause of crime. In Britain for example, government policy is increasingly to identify probation as part of an integrated criminal justice strategy including crime prevention, policing, victim support and the management of offenders (see for example Moxon 1985; Locke 1990; Harris 1992). This conjunction in turn means that a different set of principles for probation is coming to be articulated, based on public policy priorities such as the imposition of cheap, non-custodial punishment for offenders whose crimes are not deemed to justify the dedication of a costly prison place (see for example Greenwood with Abrahamse 1982; and, contentiously, Lemert 1993).

CONDITIONAL SUSPENSION OF PUNISHMENT

Probation's suspensiveness takes different forms, and discussing it will preoccupy us in Chapter 2. Suspensiveness does not mean that probation cannot *be* punishment, albeit that in its original formulation in Massachusetts in 1878 reference was made to people being 'reformed without punishment'.[1] It is widely believed that any punishment entailed in probation should at least regard rehabilitation as a desirable by-product, and in many countries probation is regarded as a means to a constructive end albeit that how the end is to be achieved is sometimes unclear.

Whether probation is defined as punishment or 'an authoritarian method of treatment' (United Nations 1951: 187), it is a strategy of control simultaneously constructive and suspensive. Its controlling characteristics are embedded in this dualism: probation is an act of kindness offered as an opportunity for reformation, but containing in its fabric the possibility of overt punishment in the event of infraction (Harris and Webb 1987). Hence, while probation offers support and encouragement to those willing to take advantage of opportunity, when faced with infraction or failure probation officers are influential in determining when undesirable behaviour becomes unacceptable. At that point it becomes their duty to initiate coercion. Intrinsic to probation, therefore, are interwoven strands of liberation and constraint (Harris 1989b): probation offers criminals an opportunity, but in a context which means that any choice open to them is heavily constrained (Raynor 1978). To decline the offer of probation is possible in some jurisdictions, though to do so is likely to have negative consequences. For many offenders probation accordingly becomes an offer hard to refuse.

It follows that a purely voluntary social service for offenders without sanction in the event of infraction would not be probation. Probation's etymology is germane: *probatio*, a noun, has the sense of 'proving oneself', while *probator* is 'an approver'; and while probation officers may in individual cases offer unconditional support on a voluntary basis – to ex-prisoners, distressed offenders who have been otherwise dealt with or people suffering marital disharmony – this is not constitutive of probation and if it was all probation officers did they would not in this definition *be* probation officers.

SUPERVISION AND GUIDANCE OR TREATMENT

Depending on contemporary ideologies the guidance or treatment entailed in probation may be psychologically or psychiatrically derived therapy, a confrontational stance based on maintaining anxiety (an approach often used with paederasts), a social skills-based approach to encouraging offenders to reject temptation (McGuire and Priestley 1985) or a low key activity reflecting precisely the etymology of 'supervision' – watching over someone, possibly in the kindliest of ways.

One way of tracing the dominant ideologies of probation is by the changing training literature. Only in Britain is this literature at all extensive, however, and even there only in the last twenty years. Until recently the literature was clinical in orientation, emphasized the problems of adolescence and presented probation officers as benign and skilled therapists sensitive to the inner turmoils of 'clients' but by no means impervious to their external disadvantages (see, successively, Le Mesurier 1935; Friedlander 1947; Glover 1949; King 1958; Monger 1964). The United Nations expressed it thus:

> The scientific foundation of probation as a method for the treatment of offenders is to be found in the contemporary sciences of human behaviour, i.e., the social, psychological and behavioural sciences, and in the application of these sciences to the problems of criminal behaviour.
>
> (United Nations 1951: 268)

The role of the probation officer, who in Britain worked primarily with adolescents, was to become an 'auxiliary ego' (see in particular Blos 1962) to augment an internal ego which, in the language of ego psychology (Freud 1937), was weakened in adolescence by a massive implosion of id. Hence the probation officer was to be a mature father figure who 'supported' the egos of youngsters whose criminality and age respectively demonstrated and explained their lack of appropriate inner controls. In the optimistic language of a 1962 report on British probation the probation officer was to establish a relationship which will, itself, be a positive influence, counteracting and modifying the ill-effects of past experiences and of irremovable factors in the present.

(Report of the Departmental Committee on the Probation Service 1962: Chapter 4)

More recently, a study of probation officers' professional reading habits (Davies 1989) reveals that the most popular book in probation officers' 'top ten' (McGuire and Priestley's *Offending Behaviour* 1985) received almost as many citations as the remaining nine put together. Since this book, subtitled *Skills and Stratagems for Going Straight*, is a practical handbook which develops an approach to offending behaviour rooted in the development of social skills (including the skill to say 'no') it seems reasonable to conclude that this approach to managing offending behaviour is widely if not exclusively used by English/Welsh probation officers.

While nothing about probation determines the nature of the officer–offender contact, probation in the UN definition necessarily involves such contact taking place as a means of ensuring the probation officer monitors, advises and helps the offender in a professionally and culturally acceptable way. Conditional freedom without such contact exists in many jurisdictions, and though it is not probation in the contemporary sense, in much of continental Europe 'probation' was originally conceptually and operationally distinct from 'supervision'. So far as we are aware, this is now seldom the case other than, for reasons we explain in Chapter 2, in the United States, where it co-exists with supervised probation.

There are other possible features of probation systems which, though not constitutive of probation, are characteristic of specific probation services. So probation officers may or may not be social workers, and may or may not be professionals: in Japan, for example, not only is the use of paraprofessional helpers widespread (see for example Hogan 1971; Gordon 1976; Terrill 1992) but the bulk of supervision is carried out by volunteers (VPOs) who, following the Volunteer Probation Officer Law 1950, number some 48,000–50,000 (Hess 1970; Nakayama 1987; Moriyama 1989; Nishikawa 1994). Indeed a 1984 study showed one probation officer on average to be responsible for 148 offenders and 80 VPOs (Rehabilitation Bureau, Ministry of Justice, Japan 1990: 11).

In Sweden too, with an integrated prison and probation administration (Nelson 1987; Terrill 1992), there are few probation officers but numerous lay supervisors, who receive only expenses and a modest honorarium. While probation officers are civil servants and university graduates normally with experience in counselling or social welfare, most supervisors lack specific qualifications but possess appropriate personal qualities and mature judgement:

> Thus a probation officer's case-load (averaging 42 clients) will include on the one hand his own supervision assignments and on the other hand assignments allocated to a lay supervisor, where the probation officer's main function is to offer guidance to the layman.
>
> (Cartledge *et al.* 1981: 412)

Probation officers in different jurisdictions may or may not advise courts on sentencing options; be involved with parole; be civil servants; work in prisons; have duties unconnected with crime such as responsibilities in connection with divorce or child custody proceedings. An offender's consent to probation may or may not have to be secured; probation may or may not be mixed with another sentence; and any permitted mixture may be concurrent or consecutive (normally with prison). In short our aim in developing a three-limbed definition of probation is not to suggest that probation officers undertake no other activities, but that even if they do not they are recognizable as probation officers if they meet our three criteria.

Probation as currently understood involves handing over an offender to expert ministration. It is hence frequently used as a flexible means of enabling courts to impose an individualized sentence in a case where a tariff punishment would offend against the canons of commonsense or common decency. Probation also permits the continual monitoring of risky offenders, enabling the system to respond pragmatically and speedily to changes in behaviour, and in some countries, particularly the United States, attempts have been made to harness the level or nature of supervision to the risk posed by the offender (see for example Clear and O'Leary 1983; McCarthy 1987; Noonan and Latessa 1987; Walker 1989; Zvekic 1994). It thus reflects not only (and sometimes only tangentially) the offence committed but also the progress of the offender. This raises long-recognized issues of civil liberties:

While modern criminal law has restricted the use of force, it has intensified the direct appeal to man's personality. If the Rule of Law is to be maintained these new tendencies require new forms of legal guarantees for man's rights and liberty. . . . The balance between the requirements of social case-work and the respect for the individual's personal rights and liberty must be drawn within the framework of each particular national legal system and socio-cultural traditions.

(United Nations 1954b: 88)

The social and philosophical concerns which stem from conjunctions of this kind are an almost universal part of the European discourse of probation (Fogel 1984). In the USA the probation service is more fully incorporated in the correctional arm of the criminal justice system (Clear and Rumgay 1992), and there is evidence that in Britain the intention is that the service shall similarly effect a transition from 'a social work agency to a *managed* criminal justice service' (Home Office 1993: Objective J).

SOME ISSUES IN COMPARATIVE SOCIAL RESEARCH

In comparative research on crime and its control it is extremely difficult to isolate even relatively and apparently independent variables – for example, prisoners' diet – and the sifting of evidence about dependent variables is consequently that much more complex. At the end of the day, therefore, it is an incautious man who could say, with Sterne, 'they order . . . this matter better in France' without hedging the statement with innumerable caveats.

(Croft 1979: 7–8)

To Croft's literary allusion, which reflects the well-established definitional difficulties in comparative research, must be added methodological differences among cross-national studies, such as variations in research designs between different countries. For example, Doleschal notes that whereas North American criminological research characteristically follows the classical hypothetico-deductive reductionist design ('two or more randomly selected groups of subjects, only one of which receives the treatment under inquiry'), in Europe the predominant mode is 'a descriptive

analysis of all available statistics and information on a given topic
... presenting the kind of data most frequently found in annual
reports of American correctional agencies' (National Institute of
Mental Health 1971: 2). Hence with few exceptions 'the student
of crime and delinquency should not expect to find, in European
research, controlled and experimental studies using rigid designs
and sociometric methods' (National Institute of Mental Health
1971: 5). Accordingly, the Netherlands excepted, to the North
American eye criminological research in Europe has traditionally
been 'generally unsatisfactory' (National Institute of Mental
Health 1971: 11).

The dominant European perspective (where the main American
criminal justice journals are read by only the specialist few)
is quite different and the conventional response to the epistemo-
logical challenge of American empiricism is to argue that the
application of sophisticated measurement tools to a sample of,
say, pre-adolescent substance abusers in New Mexico is of little
help to correctional or police workers in Marseilles or Belfast.
There the preference tends to be for a broader, less specific
knowledge-base supported by more discursive and speculative
theoretical ideas as to the possible meanings and implications
of the data.

To some positivist researchers in the social sciences, particularly
of optimistic disposition, comparative research permits a precision
of analysis and control over variables normally available to the
pure scientist, so contributing to the creation of the predictive
precision to which many American criminologists aspire:

> In the chemistry laboratory it is possible for the researcher to
> add one substance to another in a test tube, to heat to a specific
> temperature, and to observe and measure the reaction ... the
> social scientist is rarely able to manipulate the variables
> directly. With the use of the comparative method and through
> the careful selection and/or sampling of research sites, however,
> he can manipulate the experimental variables indirectly.
>
> (Holt and Turner 1970: 8)

Such a view, however, arguably skates over the many epistemo-
logical objections to such an approach (see for example Berting
1988; Scheuch 1990), understating the tactical problems which
any attempt at uncontaminated comparative research would face.
One such problem is that because one is normally dealing

with at least one foreign culture one cannot be confident that the commonsense assumptions of day-to-day life apply or that workaday categorizations are meaningful. Human adaptive capacity is stretched when, as commonly occurs, everyday conventions and attributions of causality begin to disintegrate. This applies not only to language (for a helpful discussion see Hymes 1970) but also to paralinguistic behaviour such as kinesics (the body motion aspects of human behaviour) and proxemics (the spatial contextualization of communication) (Hall 1966: Chapters XI–XII). So when one is interviewing a subject for whom a steadfast gaze does *not* signify honesty and integrity but intrusion and rudeness, for whom laughter does not mean what it commonly means in the west, or for whom a failure to anticipate the expected response is a mark of discourtesy (for a discussion of courtesy bias see Armer 1973); when one is working in a society where the words 'yes' and 'no' do not exist (though the concepts may [Hymes 1970: 301]), or where there is no way of saying 'thank you', the western researcher is liable to be brought up sharply. And, to pursue the problem a little further, if middle-class Indians ask strangers their salary much as westerners ask strangers their occupation (Grimshaw 1973: 26) it is clear that taken-for-granted categories of courtesy or rudeness differ among cultures and that money and privacy have contrasting social meanings in the west and India. Not surprisingly therefore, observed differences between societies may be artefactual not real (Armer 1973: 51), seemingly simple tools of social enquiry coming to require careful consideration and testing lest they yield unreliable data or give offence in application.

This, however, is not a problem for comparative research alone. In any interrogative encounter researchers need to be aware of the impact of their presence on the subject, of the social context in which the encounter occurs, how the research is 'read' by the subject and how the subject is likely to have been trained to deal with the encounter itself. Similarly, in any cross-cultural or cross-linguistic encounter speech communities will interact variably, and in a manner reflective of broader cultural and social relations (Gumperz 1971). Though not unique to comparative research problems such as this apply especially poignantly there, for the social interventions entailed in field study may be culturally inappropriate, while the encounter as a whole may be shrouded in suspicion, apprehension or confusion:

Why should anyone trust a snooping sociologist? In my first comparative study along the US–Mexican border, I became aware that informants in each country responded differently to the same research strategy. In subsequent comparative studies, I concluded that these differences resulted from informant distrust and that this factor varied enormously from one country to another.

(Form 1973: 83)

Another, as sensitive to the possible reputation of the United States among some respondent populations as it behoves researchers from any former colonial power to be about possible perceptions held about them, notes that:

Many US researchers combine high methodological skill with a political naiveté which makes them assume that 'good intentions' will be sufficient to dispel doubts and earn the goodwill of local scholars and citizens.

(Portes 1973: 150)

Our own approach has been to adopt a hybrid methodology. The researchers undertook no primary fieldwork themselves but sought to produce a collaborative endeavour with experts from the countries concerned, both because this was an economically feasible way to proceed and because it was preferable to translating 'native' data into the categories and concepts of our own cultures and theoretical orientations (Kohn 1989b). The term 'hybrid' is employed primarily because the method of study is mixed – a combination of discussion, the administration of a questionnaire which combines objective information with subjective (though still expert) opinion, and subsequent communication, for clarification and elaboration, with the experts responsible for questionnaire completion. This is a familiar approach for members of the research team, and this book is in part complementary to earlier studies of crimę control, policing and corrections with which one of us in particular has been involved (Findlay and Zvekic 1988; 1993; Zvekic 1994).

There is, however, a second and no less significant meaning attached to our hybridity. No levity is intended when we suggest that the multi-national character of the team, comprising Japanese, Swiss, Serbian, Welsh and English researchers, was itself a helpful corrective to any temptation to produce premature or monocultural explanations. It has more than once occurred to us that this benefit was not available to the majority of the (predominantly North American) comparative researchers cited in this section.

These general complexities were further compounded by the fact that probation is a western idea based on western administrative arrangements and assumptions. Beyond this, however, not only is it not a unitary concept even in the west but it has been imported by countries where it has been further adapted, made to overlay pre-existing formal and informal arrangements and fitted into local criminal justice systems. In Papua New Guinea for example, the Chief Probation Officer notes that in the New Guinea Islands Region:

> On many occasions, Courts requested Probation Officers to include in their Reports, the type of traditional punishment given to offenders by village elders, councillors and Village Court Magistrates. It was pleasing to see the Judges and Magistrates imposing customary forms of punishment on the Offenders. By imposing these penalties, the offender, relatives of the offender, the victim and relatives showed more appreciation to the Courts for the Orders given.
>
> (Tohichem 1991)

Theoretical and empirical questions arise as to why certain countries should import probation systems and others should not. Are there economic, cultural or political preconditions for such an importation which can be identified by conventional anthropological enquiry? Can we, by comparative political research (perhaps along the lines developed in Holt and Turner 1970) trace an imperial legacy in the cultural logic accorded probation in, for example, Papua New Guinea, Malaysia, Hong Kong or India? How can we make sense of the development, maintenance and usage of probation in Israel (intimately connected as it has historically been with Britain and the United States) and the Philippines, given its close historical connection with Spain (where no organized system of probation exists) and the USA (where probation began)?

We know that in the Philippines probation was introduced during the US administration and has followed the American model of having a firm correctional focus. Nevertheless it is used for a particular purpose: to remove short sentence prisoners from custody. As in Papua New Guinea, where the Australian influence has been considerable but not simple, probation was grafted on to a relatively recently developed system of village courts, instituted in 1975 to take over the functions of local courts to increase community support:

> The main reason Village Courts were introduced or established in Papua New Guinea, was as a dispute-settlement mechanism midway between the Western-oriented and excessively legalistic formal Court-system and the traditional localized mechanisms based on customary usage. It was set up mainly in an attempt to institutionalize the traditional dispute-settling mechanism.
>
> (Keris 1992)[2]

In Israel there is again American influence, but this overlays a native belief in psychological explanations of human behaviour which, though also striking in the USA, has not there extended to a therapeutic mode of treatment for most offenders. Indeed in their contemporary productions of probation work, Israel and the United States are at opposite poles on an axis which places probation between the extremes of treatment and correctionalism.

When to this are added the varying origins of probation and its volatility to political and economic change, it will be clear that to express the defining characteristics of probation more precisely than by the three definers identified already would be reckless. The methodological problems we face are of *conceptual equivalence*: we may be measuring the same 'thing' at a denotational but not a connotational level:

> The same word in two languages may have different connotations. .... The same sample may have a different position with respect to the total society (e.g., communities of 25,000 may be cities in some societies but towns or villages in others; 18-year-olds may be adults in some societies but not in others). The same measurement techniques in two societies may measure different aspects of reality. ... As a result of such problems, differences observed in the data for the two societies may be artifacts of method rather than valid differences.
>
> (Armer 1973: 51)

It is important to avoid reification. For all the need which exists to define probation so as to make it practically recognizable, essentialism is unhelpful. Probation is less a 'thing' to be exported or imported than a framework, broadly recognizable internationally, for dealing with criminal justice issues which are, in that place and at that time, decreed by significant definers as problems better dealt with by probation than by any other means.

Comparative researchers are themselves in dispute concerning fundamentals of their trade (see for example Øyen 1990: 5), and wide-ranging differences exist in the nature of comparative study. This is not surprising given that comparative research may embrace anything from the most minute aspect of an interpersonal encounter to the largest element of macro-political structure. This variety must raise questions as to whether, for example, the country itself is object or context, unit of analysis (the debate among anthropologists about the appropriate unit social group goes back many years – see for example Hobhouse *et al.* 1930) or part of a transnational framework which regards nations as subsystems of an international totality (Kohn 1989c: 20–4).

What constitutes comparative research is by definition dependent on the acceptance of certain assumptions about social and physical boundaries. It is not self-evident that the nation-state boundary is the most appropriate one on which to base comparative study: nations and states are by no means the same thing (for a helpful discussion of this point and an excellent typology see Oommen 1989: 201 *et seq.*; see also Finsterbusch 1973), and not only do many single country societies yield rich data for comparative study (for a discussion of cross-cultural research within India see Gumperz 1971; Elder 1973) but employing a specific boundary as the basis of comparison can be a source of misleading conclusions:

coronary heart disease has a much higher incidence in Finland than in neighbouring Sweden. An analysis of the survey data by subregion rather than only country by country showed that this high incidence was entirely due to the concentration of that ailment in the northern, much more rural half of Finland; values for the southern, more developed part – where one would otherwise expect higher incidences – were identical with rates for Sweden, Denmark and Norway. ... It was not 'Finland' as a nation-state, culture or society that could account for the odd values, but Finland as an administrative unit included a setting with aberrant living conditions.

(Scheuch 1990: 29)

For present purposes the term 'cross-institutional' probably best describes the study reported here, in that our focus is a single institution – probation – in different countries, and studying it should throw light not only on the direct object of analysis but also, because this object cannot itself be unyoked from the socio-political context in which it operates, on the meaning and structure of criminal justice and the social and natural ecology of the countries concerned.

In India, for example, competing economic priorities, the weakness of central control over the states, geography, the low status of professional help and a mismatch between offenders' problems and probation officers' imported clinical ideologies combined to render probation marginal. Nor is this phenomenon unique to India, nor specific to probation work (Rodenborg 1986; Durst 1992). In Papua New Guinea the organization of the recently formed probation service (the Probation Act 1979 was effectively implemented in 1985) was affected by diverse factors which included the transfer to other duties of sympathetic and well-informed magistrates, internal political reorganization, variable support from provincial administrations, telephone disconnections among offenders, non-availability of transport (cars and dinghies) for probation officers, the misuse of pool cars by a minority of officers and widespread tribal fighting in Enga Province, which prevented VPOs undertaking training (Tohichem 1991).

Though in the geographically larger developed countries of Australia, Canada and the United States technological supervision (by telephone or computer link) is feasible, this is not always so in developing countries where the choice is likely to be between supervision by co-opted members of the local community (an approach which itself makes assumptions about the nature of that community, the political structure and stability of the state and the relations between the two) and no supervision. In the larger countries it is possible that the impact of geography on the nature and character of probation has been under-researched: distant supervision involves fewer opportunities for group-based activities such as activity centres or community service or for relationship-building between supervisor and supervisee. This creates modes of distant supervision based on routine reporting and random, possibly technological, surveillance.

COMPARATIVE PROBATION RESEARCH

A modest tradition of both cross-country and comparative study of criminology and criminal justice exists (see for example Heidensohn and Farrell 1991; Heiland *et al.* 1991; Alvazzi del Frate *et al.* 1993; Farrington and Walklate 1993; Vagg 1993). The study of cross-country criminal justice policy, however, frequently falls into subcategories. Hence while the concerns of some researchers are with criminal justice systems as a whole (for example Cole *et al.* 1987; Terrill 1992) others have concentrated on a subset of the system – for example informal crime control (Findlay and Zvekic 1988), alternatives to custody (Clifford 1980; 1983; UNAFEI 1980; Conférence Permanente Européenne de la Probation 1983; Zvekic 1994), juvenile justice (Nyquist 1960; United Nations Social Defence Research Institute 1976; Hackler and Brockman 1980; Stewart 1982; Klein 1984), the death penalty (Hood 1989) or policing (Mawby 1990; Findlay and Zvekic 1993).

Very few cross-national accounts of probation exist (the main example is Cartledge *et al.* 1981) but there is a literature, albeit of variable currency and quality, on probation in different countries. This includes probation in Belgium (Versele 1969), China (Allen 1987), Denmark (Brydensholt 1980), the former German Democratic (Falkowski-Tucker 1990) and Federal Republics (Spiess and Johnson 1980), Hong Kong (Lee 1972), India (Shah 1974; Bhattacharyya 1980; 1986; Singh, D. 1980; Sahay 1981; Jeyasingh 1982; Singh, M. 1987; Srivastava 1987; Tandon 1988; Chakrabarti 1992), Israel (Reifen 1969; Tadanir 1969; Bensinger 1982; 1984; Frishtik 1988; 1991; Cohen *et al.* 1991; Nalla and Newman 1991), Italy (Breda and Ferracuti 1980), Jamaica (McBean 1972), Netherlands (Heijder 1972; Nuyten-Edelbroek and Tigges 1980; Junger-Tas and Tigges 1982; Woelinga 1990), New Zealand (Webb 1982; Pratt 1990; Eskridge and Newbold 1993), Nigeria (Milner 1972), Poland (Walczak 1969; 1976), Sweden (Edholm and Bishop 1983; Rouse 1985) and the USA (where, in addition to numerous journal articles and works cited elsewhere, recent books include Bartollas 1985; Allen *et al.* 1985; Clear and Cole 1986; Abadinsky 1991).

In spite of the limitations of our database in cross-national probation *research*, however, in the world of probation *practice* overseas influences have from the first existed (Grünhut 1948;

Bochel 1976; Page 1992) and borrowings across systems seem destined to increase within the European Union and beyond. If, however, importation occurs without theoretical underpinning there is a danger of assuming that probation has an agreed meaning which translates unproblematically into other organizational arrangements and professional practices. Any such view would be erroneous. It should be noted in particular that in spite of great differences between the British and US probation systems (Clear and Rumgay 1992) ideological as well as linguistic similarities at a level of organization and management make such borrowings rather attractive (see for example Fielder 1992; Saiger 1992).

The comparative study of different systems or subsets of systems on a cross-national basis is technically difficult. At its most basic level 'comparative' is sometimes used to classify work which comprises descriptions of systems in specific countries, normally provided by native academics or practitioners. Such accounts (following Klein 1984) we term the *first phase* in comparative analysis: the provision of descriptive data which, if accurate, comprehensive and current, may constitute a baseline for later more sophisticated analyses. Such studies must be treated cautiously, however, for not all are exemplary in their accuracy, comprehensiveness and currency, and some may misuse terms or use them in a particularistic, undefined and misleading way (for a discussion of this problem in comparative research see Vagg 1993).

The researcher who lacks access to, and an informed awareness of, all contemporary materials in any country to which reference is made is in the hands of studies most readily available. This is undesirable and may lead to false attributions and conclusions, yet to proceed only when in possession of perfect data would be a counsel of unattainable perfection which would consign comparative study to the scrapheap. As one researcher has wryly observed:

> One of the central research strategies, although not much discussed, seems to be the preference given to available data and methodological tools, and the leaning towards accessible networks and easy funding. The pristine goal of sociological research as a guiding principle for our choices in cross-national research may for most of us have to stay pristine.
>
> (Øyen 1990: 15)

Large-scale funding for a comparative probation study would be difficult to secure, and anyway unless handled with extreme care large-scale research can conceal as much as it reveals, for 'cases lose their identities as they are disaggregated into variables' (Ragin 1989: 60). Or as one decisive commentator on probation expressed it, in relation to predictive measures:

> standard methods give birth to fictional characteristics of types which are superimposed upon the real characteristics or type of a certain person. To know that disaffection, hostility, rejection, etc., appear in the majority of cases is not of particular help for probation and parole purposes. What is important is the particular kind of rejection, hostility, disaffection, etc., in each individual case.
>
> (López-Rey 1957: 348)

Even the more modest aim of drawing together existing comparative and cross-national studies in our field is, however, not straightforward: much of the literature antedates computerized databases and much of it is anecdotal and descriptive, for probation has been a major focus of empirical study only where it is most developed. The choice, therefore, is between inadequate comparative study and no comparative study. The process of peer correction, updating and development which leads to a secure tradition is a long one and it is appropriate to our present level of knowledge to engage in what has been termed the logic of discovery (the reasons for entertaining a hypothesis) not of proof (the reasons for accepting one) (Kaplan 1964). To create what Kaplan terms a 'pattern' for more definitive subsequent work which will, if all goes well, repudiate or transform beyond recognition our preliminary efforts reasonably states our present ambition.

The *second phase* of cross-national/comparative study is the juxtaposition of different systems. Juxtaposition entails creating and utilizing a systematic methodology to increase the robustness of data. In this book such a methodology exists: it entails selecting research areas, identifying an expert from each country, creating a questionnaire, meeting the experts after a draft response has been prepared, refining the instrument and giving respondents time to develop or reconsider their answers, liaising on points of ambiguity or difficulty – and in the wake of all this producing a report. This hybrid method is consistent with other studies of social phenomena which have addressed the impossibility of attaining detailed understanding by macro-analysis or irrefutable proof by micro-analysis by developing an approach close to our own:

> If we wait ... until every step of the way has been cleared by microstudies, a millenium would hardly suffice. To fill the vast gap in between, what seems to be developing in comparative studies is a composite method that combines the use of documentation, aggregate data, secondary analysis and reliance on strategic individual researches at the field level. The compound results of these efforts have advanced our knowledge of total society functioning which microanalysis by itself cannot attain.
>
> (Schermerhorn 1970: 253)

From this a *third phase* is possible and we do not claim to have a secure bolt hole there. This entails 'a conceptual analysis based upon comparative descriptions' (Klein 1984: 14). We have begun this conceptual work by identifying key aspects of probation such as function, status, professionalization, training, the use of volunteers, and both *comparing* the way in which these aspects exist in the case study countries and beginning to *theorize* the concepts themselves to offer a possible meaning – or multiplicity of meanings – of what is constitutive of probation round the world.

CONCLUSION

This chapter has sought to set the scene for what follows, referring only briefly to some of the countries included in the study. The Editors' Introduction invited readers to develop what, modifying C. Wright Mills's concept of the sociological imagination, we termed a comparative imagination. This makes two distinct intellectual demands. The first is to make a cognitive shift which involves decentring one's own professional preoccupations. This shift in turn has two main dimensions: to problematize what one does unthinkingly by exposing it to the possibility that other people in other systems do and perceive the same things equally unthinkingly but differently; and to 'locate' oneself as part of a large, variegated enterprise relevant to one's own activities. In short one comes to grasp a certain relevance to one's own activities of those of probation workers round the world, and from this grasp comes a personal repositioning of a perceptual and strategic kind.

The second demand is the converse of this. One of the theoretical axes on which all comparative research turns is that of similarity and difference. This surfaces most explicitly in this chapter in the gap between micro-level research (which, by using single or small number case design, highlights detailed differences between people, groups or small systems) and macro-level research which offers broad patterns, theoretically comprehensible as a generality but with deviations from the norm seldom effectively analysed or explained.

Our concern in inviting a comparative imagination is not to suggest unities which do not exist: it is as far from our theoretical interests to minimize 'difference' in comparative study as it would be in single country research. Certainly we hope to establish sufficient commonality among professionals to breed a sense of underlying collegiality and mutual interest, but then to use this sense as a basis for exploring points of difference as well as similarity. We have tried too, however, to indicate some of the problems, tactical and conceptual, involved in such an enquiry. This book, because it has no secure tradition of cross-national probation research on which to draw, is primarily exploratory and, inevitably, tentative. Accordingly its longer term usefulness may lie less in its theorization of data than in its existence as a starting point for more ambitious studies. We hope, however, that it will create interest and stimulate debate within probation and criminal justice's academic and professional communities, to whom it is likely that our subject matter will become of more rather than less interest in the years ahead.

NOTES

1 This point is fully discussed, albeit with contrary conclusions drawn, in United Nations 1951: 185–8 and Harris 1989b. It is also of note that it was also envisaged by the Massachusetts Statute of 1878 that the supervisor should be a police officer, or at least under the supervision of the chief of police in Boston – though this arrangement was quickly reversed.

2 It is important to note that the assumption that 'customary law' comprised a truly indigenous pre-colonial form of justice administration on to which western forms have been subsequently grafted has been subjected to strong theoretical attack. For the suggestion that 'customary law' is itself an ideological weapon of colonialism see Snyder 1982; for accounts of the PNG village court and dispute resolution systems see Paliwala 1982 and Fitzpatrick 1982.

Chapter 2

Probation round the world
Origins and development

Robert Harris

... the facts that we have to explain are pretty much similar in most societies. Crime is perpetrated disproportionately by males, by young persons, and by persons living in cities. Stronger attachment to school, higher levels of educational attainment, and strong familial relationships are contra-indications for criminality. High mobility, poverty, and close relationships with other offenders are all associated with offending. Yet the extent to which, in any given society, there are linkages between juvenile and youth crime and – for example – adult-oriented organized crime must make a difference not just to the kinds of theories we might consider, but to the more fundamental question of what it is we are trying to explain.

(Vagg 1993: 545–6)

Some problems would not be problems if they presented themselves on the other side of the border, or at least they might be problems of a different kind.

(Lorenz 1994: 170)

Probation round the world has its origins in two distinct traditions, common and civil (or statute) law. Though these traditions have converged in the post-World War Two period and have little explanatory power today, traces of them are periodically discernible in probation's literature and discourse. Hence, in this field certainly but doubtless also as a general principle, an historical perspective is necessary if the present is to be even imperfectly comprehended.

The traditions serve also as a heuristic device for exposing certain tensions widespread in probation round the world. Some of these tensions emerge explicitly, others implicitly in this chapter. They include the definition of and relation between care and control, the place of discretion and individualism as opposed to legalism in criminal justice, the impact of offending on citizenship rights and the regenerative as against repressive purposes of criminal justice (for considerations of this kind of issue see Fielding 1984; Raynor 1985; May 1991).

The contours of the relation between the traditions reveal an increasing convergence *between* them, but increasing diversification *within* them. On the one hand interpenetration has occurred, provoking a convergence, the civil law countries of continental Europe softening their formalism in the light of the achievements of the Anglo-Saxon tradition and the common law countries introducing legislative changes which render probation's statutory basis increasingly explicit. Yet alongside this convergence has come a greater heterogeneity within traditions. So though we categorize England and Wales,[1] the United States and the Old Commonwealth countries as representative of the common law tradition, probation in these countries has developed very differently. This is partly because in a number of common law countries informality has come into conflict with constitutional rights, and partly because probation has proved sufficiently malleable to assume characteristics which ensure its relevance to local problems.

Among civil law countries differences exist in relation to the adoption of common law practices, the role of voluntary organizations, particularly the Church, and the co-option as supervisors of members of the community. This latter tendency has been a strong element in Danish and Swedish probation, but assumes particular significance in those parts of Eastern Europe where a collectivist tradition led, in the years following the Russian Revolution, to the introduction of community supervision by youth and trade union organizations, families and workmates.

We shall refer to this collectivist tradition in Hungary later in the book; particularly striking, however, was a practice in the former Czechoslovakia, where an Act of 1919, while following the Franco-Belgian system of suspending sentence (United Nations 1951: 79) did so by assigning to probationers as a protective supervisor a *duverník* (a confidential friend or shop steward), a *porucník* (a supervising tutor for those aged under 21, who might be a relative of the offender) or an *opatrovník* (a trustee or guardian for adults) (Trought 1927: 47). It fell to these supervisors to report periodically to the court on the offender's progress.

Germany following reunification also offers an interesting if incomplete case study of probation's necessary relation to the dominant political structure. Reunification brought many economic, legal and practical problems for probation officers in the former Federal Republic (Falkowski-Tucker 1990). In the former Democratic Republic probation had been available as a sentence since 1968, but based on the collectivist system of workplace supervision by volunteers, with discharged prisoners guaranteed employment and accommodation. These guarantees disappeared with the political and economic turbulence and rapidly rising crime rate which accompanied reunification. Attempts were made by the Federal German service to advise on instituting probation in the East, but in spite of the successful introduction of probation to the Eastern *land* of Sachsen-Anhalt in 1991 probation had low priority among many more necessary investments. In particular the political, personal and professional unsuitability of former GDR personnel to continue following reunification meant that a new system with new personnel had to be constructed almost *ab initio* (Falkowski-Tucker 1990; Wegener 1991).

The dramatic changes in the Democratic Republic demonstrate the extent to which probation draws for its social, political and professional meaning on the ideological context of time as well as place. Probation is vulnerable to political change because much of what appears its essence is a social and political artefact; hence in Eastern Europe arrangements which sufficed in the former Democratic Republic took on such different political and economic meanings following reunification as to render them impossible.

The transformation of a sentence rooted in western Enlightenment philosophy into a collectivist mode of supervision illustrates probation's capacity to dovetail into existing arrangements in a manner appropriate to a particular time and place. This capacity will re-emerge throughout this analysis as a strong characteristic of probation round the world.

THE COMMON LAW TRADITION

> Once a person got into trouble through drink or any other
> crime there seemed no hope. Offence after offence, and
> sentence after sentence appeared to be the inevitable lot of
> him whose foot had once slipped ... could nothing be done
> to arrest the downward career?
>
> (Ayscough 1923: 12)

> the probation officer should learn to be more than an individual
> virtuoso.
>
> (Parsloe 1969: 99)

United States of America

In Britain and much of North America the origins of probation
lie in the mediaeval common law practices of releasing offenders
on recognizance (or 'binding them over') on condition that they
were of good behaviour and kept the peace, and the surety system
of bail release.[2] In the recognizance system imported to America
by the early settlers no supervision or monitoring was involved,
though localized forms of voluntary supervision were sometimes
associated with it. The surety system on the other hand made a
willing third party responsible for producing an offender in court,
penalizing him/her financially if he/she failed to do so.

It was as a confluence of these traditions that probation
emerged, being first 'named' by a Boston shoemaker, John
Augustus (1785–1859) (United Nations 1951; Chute and Bell 1956;
Diana 1970). Working with the Washington Total Abstinence
Society Augustus began visiting the Boston police court in 1841
to undertake pre-trial enquiries, initially in respect of drunken,
but later of more diverse offenders. In the light of these enquiries
he would request a deferral of sentence in suitable cases, with the
offender committed to his care. During this period of being 'bailed
on probation' he would provide his charges with practical support
and, at the end of the deferral, accompany the offender to court,
where in successful cases by convention or agreement a nominal
sentence would be imposed. During his first ten years:

> a total of 1,102 persons were received on his bail, divided as
> follows: 674 males and 428 females, 569 from the Police Court
> and 533 from the Municipal Court; 116 boys under sixteen.

The total amount of bail pledged was $99,464. Fines and costs paid (mostly by defendants) were $2,417.65. Up to 1858, one year before his death, he had put up bail for 1,946 persons.

(Chute and Bell 1956: 44)

After Augustus's death his work was carried on by Haskins, a priest who worked to reform some 3,000 boys until his death in 1872 and Cook, a house painter, prison chaplain and first agent of the Children's Aid Society, who claimed in 1870 to have bailed 450 people of all ages.

The first Probation Act,[3] enacted in Massachusetts in 1878, provided for the appointment by the Mayor of Boston of a paid probation officer (the first was Police Lieutenant Henry C. Hemmenway), and specified that probation was to enable people to be 'reformed without punishment'. The Act vested no new powers in courts but envisaged punishment for violators arrested by the probation officer on police authority. Amending legislation of 1880 and 1881, however, severed the link between probation and police, and an Act of 1891 transferred powers of appointment from the municipality to the courts, making such appointments mandatory at lower court level throughout the state. By 1898 this duty had extended to superior courts, and when in 1900 probation was given a statutory basis in judicial sentencing procedures it ceased to be available solely prior to sentence, coming also to accompany a suspension of its execution.

This step was taken partly with the practical aim of permitting the simultaneous execution of one sentence and suspension of another, so that fines imposed alongside probation could be collected by probation officers (Chute and Bell 1956: 66). Of equal significance, however, was a challenge to the legality of suspending sentences issued by Attorney-General Gregory in 1915. This provoked defiance from the legal profession, and to secure an authoritative determination of judicial powers of suspension a case in which Judge Killits, following tradition not statute, had passed a prison sentence suspended for five years was chosen for Supreme Court adjudication. The Supreme Court's unanimous judgement, handed down by Chief Justice White in 1916, was that irrespective of common law tradition suspension was unconstitutional. The judgement, however, stressed that it was the wish of the court to structure not abolish judicial discretion (Chute and Bell 1956: 97; Dressler 1969: 32), and accordingly a lengthy campaign ensued for probation with suspension.[4] A federal probation law was finally passed in 1925.

Though it emerged from British common law therefore, American probation early assumed characteristics which distanced it from its original humanitarian mission, rendered it consonant with a cultural character in which caring for criminals was less acceptable than in those continental European countries where social explanations of crime predominated and imbued it, for constitutional reasons, with a firmer statutory basis. On the other hand, American probation was and is insufficiently systematic for any approach based on consistency and fairness to exist. It has developed piecemeal, its units of organization range through city and town, county, state and federal government, its functions and duties vary widely.

> Often one agency may be required to serve juvenile, misde-meanant, and felony offenders. But while some agencies handle all three types, others handle these offenders separately. The term 'probation' has multiple meanings within the multiple areas of corrections
>
> (Allen and Simonsen 1978: 162)

> The fragmented nature of U.S. probation systems is difficult to overstate. In all major cities of the United States, there is more than one probation agency in operation, and sometimes there are as many as three with distinct legal jurisdictions covering the same geographical area . . . There is no single U.S. 'service' – indeed, many observers would object to the use of the word service to describe probation.
>
> (Clear and Rumgay 1992: 4)

Nevertheless there do exist some defining characteristics of US probation today.

- With 55 per cent of the US correctional population on proba-tion, it, not prison, is today's sentence of choice.
- Probation need not be accompanies by supervision.
- Probation officers have generally lower status than their British counterparts; their training varies widely, they have little connection with social work or social reform, and their claim for professional status is tenuous.
- Though much US probation has a correctional orientation geared to law enforcement, tensions and perceptions of role

conflict continue to exist, particularly for female staff, who studies show to be overall less punitive than their male counterparts (Whitehead 1989; Whitehead and Lindquist 1992; Silverman 1993).

- Studies of intensive supervision programmes suggest that tight control without a social support orientation is less effective than strategies which seek to combine the two (Byrne *et al.* 1989; Petersilia and Turner 1991). Hence psychologically protective distancing strategies designed to reduce role strain may be undesirable.

- Stress has resulted from the fact that as elsewhere today's probation caseload includes many more serious offenders than hitherto (Petersilia *et al.* 1985; Petersilia 1987; Lindner and Koehler 1992). This in turn has:

  § focused discussion on the home visit system: home visits are most likely to be ordered in respect of high risk offenders but involve the greatest risk of violence (Lindner 1992);
  § triggered a debate as to whether officers should be permitted or required to carry guns. Sixty-five per cent of US probation districts permit probation officers to be armed (Brown 1990); of a sample of 159 probation officers, 59 per cent favoured carrying firearms, and 80 per cent would not object to doing so if so instructed (Sluder *et al.* 1991).

- The decentralized nature of US probation has led to considerable resource pressures in some jurisdictions, and a lack of effective monitoring of standards. These problems have contributed to maintaining the relatively low status of US probation. For example:

  § caseloads are very high by international standards – the average New York City probation officer's caseload in the 1980s was 225 while in Los Angeles the figure was up to 1,000. In Nassau County New York numbers increased by 25 per cent in the period 1981–8 (Lindner 1992);
  § there have been widespread experiments with a fee system, two-thirds of US probation authorities collecting fees from probationers, sometimes on a commission basis, with fee revenue covering anything between 1 and 60 per cent of agency budgets (Wheeler *et al.* 1989; Finn and Parent 1993). While this system is consonant with a culture of

individualism, and some fees have been justified in therapeutic as well as financial terms this appears more a *post
hoc* rationalization than the prime mover of the fee system.

England and Wales

The origins of probation can be traced to the 1820s, when
Warwickshire magistrates combined the common law surety and
recognizance systems by releasing young offenders into the charge
of an employer. A step in the direction of formalization was taken
when, as Recorder of Birmingham from 1839 to 1865, Matthew
Davenport Hill, who had had first-hand experience of the Warwickshire system, began releasing young offenders into the
guardianship of members of the community. Hill's practices of
using a 'confidential officer' to make periodic enquiries, and
of keeping a record of whom he had released and how they had
fared in order that repeat offenders could be dealt with especially
firmly was an early step towards bureaucratizing probation
(Grünhut 1948: 299; United Nations 1951: 16–23, 43–7; King 1958:
1–2; Bochel 1976: 4–5; Page 1992: 6).

English probation is normally regarded as beginning in 1876
(McWilliams 1983) when Rainer, a Hertford printer, approached
Canon Ellison, Chairman of the Church of England Temperance
Society, to suggest extending the Society's activities to police courts
to offer practical help to alcoholic offenders. The suggestion was
quickly acted upon and the first missionary, Nelson, was appointed
to Southwark Police Court on 1 August 1876 (Page 1992: 2). By
1880 there were 4 missionaries in the London police courts, and at
the time of the Probation of Offenders Act 1907 143 missionaries
were at work, including 19 women (Page 1992: 56; for a first-hand
if florid account of the work of the missionaries see Holmes 1900).
Invariably the system involved supervision being offered in lieu
of sentence.

The Probation of Offenders Act 1907, which statutorily distinguished probation from binding over, maintained the missionary
tradition by permitting a probation order to be made, with consent
and following the establishment of guilt, 'without proceeding to
conviction' in a court of summary jurisdiction, and 'in lieu of
imposing a sentence of imprisonment' in a superior court. Though
this former rather subtle formulation was described in 1919 by
Mr Justice Darling as 'merely a concession to the modern passion

for calling things what they are not, for finding people guilty and
at the same time trying to declare them not guilty' (cited in United
Nations 1951: 195)[5] it is important to understand that the development of probation in England was associated with suspending
the imposition not the execution of sentence.

The widespread disillusionment with the austere uniform penal
theories of the nineteenth century (Fox 1952: 48–56) reflected both
popular humanitarian concern for the poor and a belief that
prisons were contaminating and therefore counterproductive. It
was these inefficiencies as much as any collective act of kindness
which drove the moves towards the individualization necessary
for the introduction and development of probation.

In supervised probation, individualization occurs in two ways.
First, at the point of sentence a judicial selection, professionally
guided and based on moral as well as legal criteria occurs;
and second, the course of the disposal is characterized by individualization: in the language of the Probation of Offenders Act
1907 probation officers advise, assist and befriend the offender,
but they also monitor, instruct and report. Because supervised
probation involves monitoring offenders' conduct outside the
institution it is, as the civil law theorists were acutely aware, an
imposition of executive power. Strategies such as probation make
it possible to insert the control of the state into the criminal's
home, workplace or community and, because this insertion is done
by a suspension of punishment, it is barely credible that it will be
other than attractive to the criminal. Yet supervision is normally
a lesser penalty than classical justice decrees that the criminal
deserves. Accordingly failure or refusal provokes a decisive
penalty, and the greater the gap between probation supervision
and desert the greater that penalty is liable to be. Hence it has
been claimed that ironically probation's power lies in its merciful
suspensiveness (Harris and Webb 1987) and, in any analysis
of the spread of probation, that:

> one runs the risk of positing as the principle of greater leniency
> in punishment processes of individualization that are rather one
> of the effects of the new tactics of power.
>
> (Foucault 1977: 23)

In Britain therefore, probation entailed the suspension not
of a sentence already imposed but of the act of passing sentence,
and its essential character lay as much in its suspensiveness as

in its supervisory tactics. Probation is contiguous to both control and altruism, the ambiguity of this location being precisely captured in the word 'reform'. Reform involves (literally) 're-shaping' the individual; it has desirable moral connotations, offers an alternative to the rigours of prison *and* triggers a return to those rigours in the event of infraction. Thus probation appeals to a theological, literary or psychological 'grasp' of the unfulfilled potential of deprived, oppressed or evil people whose self-interest it also addresses by offering them a gateway to a better life. Nevertheless this characteristic of the common law supervisory tradition co-exists with the enforcement of sanction if the opportunity be not taken. Hence probation, in both legitimating and necessitating the continued existence of suspensive punishment:

> may involve protecting or enhancing rights which have not been enforced by other agencies; reminding people of their own social and legal duties and of the sanctions which will be enforced if they continue in dereliction of those duties; making judgements about the point at which the state should intervene compulsorily; acting to ward off as long as is proper the necessity of such compulsion; and initiating the compulsion when it is necessary or desirable to do so.
>
> (Harris 1989a: 8)

Though doubtless probation involves no conspiracy to bring the dissolute proletariat under disciplinary surveillance, recent trends in Britain and America in the intensive supervision of high risk offenders (see for example Noonan and Latessa 1987; Walker 1989; McCarthy 1987; Byrne 1990; Morris and Tonry 1990; Armstrong 1991; McCarthy and McCarthy 1991; Brownlee and Joanes 1993; Blomberg and Lucken 1994) rest uneasily with the view that any analysis of probation as subtle control can be abandoned because, quite simply:

> probation, in large part, has become a dumping ground or cheap waste disposal for cases that are not deemed worthy or affordable for punitive processing, or any other kind, for that matter.
>
> (Lemert 1993: 460)

Australia

The influence of the traditional British reformist tradition has been considerable in Old Commonwealth countries and Israel. Of some of these countries we write in greater detail in Part II, and those mentioned here which appear also as case study countries are considered only in relation to the nature and extent of their adherence to the common or civil law tradition. In Australia:

- legislation to permit the conditional release on recognizance of first or marginal offenders was enacted in all six self-governing colonies prior to the establishment of the Commonwealth of Australia in 1901. Normally there was no supervision, but where there was it was usually undertaken by police officers;
- remarkably Queensland shifted from common to civil law practice in 1886–7 in a move which anticipated by two years the introduction of the *sursis* in Belgium. Queensland was, however, influenced by the draft French law (the *loi Bérenger*) which as we shall see later inspired the Belgian law:

   The most important innovation ... was the substitution, by Queensland (followed by most of the other colonies), of the suspension of the *execution* of sentence for the suspension of the *imposition* of sentence – an innovation which seems to have been introduced quite accidentally.

   (United Nations 1951: 53)

- nevertheless probation was slow to develop. In New South Wales, for example, though provision for probation had existed since 1924 a professional service (of six officers) was only instituted in 1951 (Keefe 1972). The influence of European positivism was not strong, nor was the paternalistic notion of professional care consonant with the 'frontiersman' culture of early twentieth-century white Australia. Accordingly:

   adult probation in Australia has not developed into an official, full-time, professional service and considerable reliance has continued to be placed on the services of volunteers and/or of the agents of voluntary organizations.

   (United Nations 1951: 54)

Canada

As we shall see later, probation had a similarly slow start in Canada.

- An Act based on the British Probation of First Offenders Act 1887 came into force in 1889 and was extended in 1901; federal provision for probation supervision followed in 1921 and the law was consolidated in the Criminal Code of 1927.

- This Code permitted the release on recognizance of a first offender convicted of an offence punishable by no more than two years' imprisonment or, with the agreement of counsel for the Crown, of a more serious first offender or a second offender.
- No restrictions were placed on the recognizance period; though courts were empowered to order supervision to take place during the probation period the inextricable association between probation and supervision characteristic of Britain did not exist.
- Provincial legislation permitting the appointment of probation officers was adopted in Ontario in 1922 and British Columbia in 1946. Even there, however, an effective system did not begin until 1951 and in spite of a recommendation of the Royal Commission to Investigate the Penal System of Canada (1938) that a probation service staffed by trained social workers should be extended to the country as a whole, no such service existed elsewhere in the Dominion.
- Where it existed probation was restricted to the larger conurbations, caseloads were high and the number of officers was, in the absence of records, estimated at twenty (United Nations 1951: 60). Where no probation officer was available supervision was undertaken by police officers, sheriffs or court officials.
- As late as the 1950s it is estimated that no more than about 1,500 people were placed on probation in any year – less than 3 per cent of offenders. At a time when in a number of European countries the probation population was outstripping the prison population (United Nations 1954b) prisons were used sixteen times more frequently than probation; 60 per cent of probation orders were made in three large urban counties in Ontario (Jaffary 1949).

In both Australia and Canada, as we shall see in Part II, recent developments in probation have been dramatic, and in both countries probation has found a culturally consonant home less as a caring or therapeutic agency than as an instrument of community punishment.

India

Though the concept if not the actuality of probation was introduced early into India, probation has failed to develop into a responsive system. This results from a combination of financial, cultural, racial and geographical difficulties, lack of political will and agreement as to what role probation should play in the criminal justice system. Doubtless related to these problems Indian probation has suffered from its dependence on an imported psychiatric paradigm of practice which can scarcely begin to address the problems faced by Indian society in general or Indian offenders in particular.

* As early as 1923 the amended Code of Criminal Procedure permitted the release of minor first offenders for up to three years on 'probation of good conduct' but without provision for supervision. In emulation of British common law the system involved release on recognizance subject to returning for sentence when called on and to being of good behaviour and keeping the peace. Thus probation was introduced first, and supervision followed as resources permitted, politics decreed or experience suggested (United Nations 1951: 88).
* In 1931 an All-India Probation Bill was introduced but not enacted as a result of internal political disturbances. A government direction of 1934 ordered provincial governments to enact probation legislation, and statutory provision for probation (with or without supervision) followed in Madhya Pradesh and Madras (1936) and Uttar Pradesh and Bombay (1938). By 1951, however, only Madras had probation supervision on a province-wide basis. The Probation of Offenders Act 1958 further demanded provincial legislation, and designating 1971 Probation Year was an attempt to promote probation as an alternative to custody. Nevertheless it remains very patchy:

   > Generally, probation is regarded as an unimportant subject and in case of paucity of funds, the axe falls on the probation service ... there is a feeling in some quarters that probation is an ordinary function which any lay man can do without any special aptitude and training.
   >
   > (Bhattacharyya 1986: 70)

* Bhattacharyya (1986) and others paint a gloomy picture of probation in India today:

§ pay and status are low (though salaries vary considerably among states, those in Karnataka being more than twice those in Uttar Pradesh);

§ there is no career structure or uniform training. In the absence of an Indian training literature (Mandal 1989; Nagpaul 1993) so strong is the imported psychiatric influence on training that a probation team can without irony be described as a 'mobile laboratory' (Bhattacharyya 1986: 169). This emphasis is daily belied by the economic marginality of probationers, few of whom are in steady employment, over half of whom are illiterate (or 'literate without formal education'), and many of whom are unmarried men with low incomes:

> the majority of the probationers in West Bengal are illiterate, unmarried, rural people coming from inferior family background. Furthermore they are unskilled labourers having inadequate or self-supporting income.
>
> (Chakrabarti 1992: 121)

§ culture, tradition and geography as well as poverty conspire against escaping this clinical paradigm, in spite of the practical acknowledgement by many of the insufficiency of taking a psychiatric approach to the work:

> The success of probation is largely linked up with the effective use of community resources. While the individual support given by the probation officer in an offender's individual and emotional problems using psychiatric and psychological theories is important, it is increasingly realised that the community-based resources such as the family, schools, neighbourhood, etc., have a great deal to contribute to offenders' successful reintegration in society.
>
> (Bhattacharyya 1986: 98)

§ similar obstacles exist to creating a coherent probation system.

– In West Bengal the intention of the Probation of Offenders Act 1958 that the probation agency should use voluntary agencies to supervise probationers failed to materialize because no voluntary bodies existed (Chakrabarti 1992).

- The competence of state officers to offer effective supervision is questionable: in West Bengal only one in thirty has specialized correctional knowledge or qualifications (Chakrabarti 1992).
- The lack of available transport for probation officers prevents effective contact with offenders (Bhattacharyya 1986). As recently as 1990 in West Bengal one probation officer was required to cover up to 5,000 km^2 (Chakrabarti 1992).

New Zealand

New Zealand was the first country to emulate the Massachusetts experiment.

- Provision was made for appointing probation officers in the Probation of First Offenders Act 1886. The Offenders Probation Act 1920 confirmed probation as a judicial disposition in its own right, with offenders who breached their conditions liable to be sentenced for the original offence, separately for the breach itself, or both. The Act also gave probation officers wide-ranging powers by permitting additional requirements such as forbidding association with individuals or classes of person and approving employment arrangements.
- The first post-1920 probation officers were police officers, prison officials, voluntary officers of the Salvation Army and a few part-time paid officers. In 1926, however, the country was divided into four probation districts, each with a full-time officer and an associate probation committee comprising suitable volunteers 'representative of all classes of the community and the various religious denominations' (United Nations 1951: 134). Stipendiary officers were appointed in Auckland, Christchurch, Dunedin and Wellington, but even as late as the 1950s there were full-time officers only in the main cities, with most probation work still undertaken by police officers.
- The great growth in probation followed its redesignation as supervision by the Criminal Justice Act 1985. It thereafter developed rapidly as part of the community correction service, a centralized system divided into thirty-six districts in four regions, with 710 staff of whom 420 are probation officers responsible for supervision, parole, pre-sentence reports, community service and community care. Officers are esteemed by

courts with up to 82 per cent of sentencing recommendations taken up (Eskridge and Newbold 1993) though, consistent with the trend in other Old Commonwealth countries (for Canada see Hylton 1981; Hatt 1985; Ekstedt and Griffiths 1988; for Australia see Leivesley 1986) the service's rehabilitative framework has been replaced by 'broking' activities; it no longer has sole responsibility for the supervision of offenders but is empowered (under section 53 of the 1985 Act) to refer offenders to community-based organizations. Hence:

> current trends in legislation demand a much broader framework of intervention and a marked shift away from what remains of the old therapeutic tradition – the casework approach – as being the fulcrum of probation intervention.
> (Pratt 1990: 110)

All the main common law probation countries have seen developments of this kind in the late twentieth century, as probation has been transformed from a reformist enterprise to a variably integrated component of non-custodial penal policy. These developments have been greeted very differently in different countries. In the Netherlands, for example, where the service contains elements of both common and civil law traditions, the probation discourse contains a strong dimension of social criticism, as does that of the Israeli service. In the large and heavily unionized English and Welsh service probation officers now have responsibility for paroled or otherwise early released prisoners, community service orders and more serious offenders whom government wishes to maintain in the community in conditions of structured and conditional freedom. The controversies about this role have been considerable, as probation has been encouraged to embrace a range of new disciplinary technologies to make punishment in the community a serious policy option.

The controversy is explained by the fact that in England and Wales rank-and-file probation ideologies remain libertarian, client centred and 'anti-oppressive', while the job itself has become more control oriented. Not surprisingly therefore, part at least of the dispute between probation officers and government has focused on the possible introduction of electronic monitoring. While probation's professional press contains repeated objections to the introduction of 'tagging' schemes and some pleasure at the inconclusive-to-negative results of a government-funded pilot scheme (Mair and Nee 1990), the fact that electronic monitoring has been introduced elsewhere with approbation has passed relatively unnoticed.

South Australia, for example, has responded very differently to the new correctionalism. There electronic monitoring has been successfully implemented both for bailees and as an early release scheme, and is available on application to the Department of Correctional Services. It is accompanied by conditions of behaviour which would be unthinkably strict to English and Welsh probation staff, including abstention from drugs and alcohol under any circumstances (offenders are called in for random urine tests and committed to prison if the tests are positive or if they fail to report) and a prohibition on gambling, taking a loan or driving a car or motor cycle without the supervisor's approval (Department of Correctional Services 1987).

An innovation such as electronic monitoring cannot be 'read' in an essentialist way. It *becomes* something different in probation round the world because it impacts variably on prevailing professional cultures and values. In England and Wales the discussion about electronic monitoring is not only about its reductionist efficacy, its economics or its success in ensuring bailees appear in court, but also about whether it is compatible with probation as probation officers perceive it to be: in this way probation's traditions affect its present behaviour. In an organization as heavily normative as the English and Welsh service those traditions overlie any legislative and ideological changes imposed from outside.

The gradual toughening of probation in Britain means that the transformation of probation into a sentence (under the Criminal Justice Act 1991) only gave statutory recognition to what had been *de facto* reality for some time. It necessitated other shifts: for probation-as-sentence to be acceptable to courts, minimum standards had to be established – as they have in other Old Commonwealth countries – specifying contact frequency minima and procedures for managing misconduct. The idea that responsibility for determining the proper response to infraction should be based on professional expertise and values, though seen as inevitable and progressive in the 1950s, inexorably gave way to a return to legalism and due process and therefore to the relocation of responsibility for detailed decision-making into the courts. In no common law country can probation any longer be considered a common law disposal.

THE CIVIL LAW TRADITION

Society may legally punish and, in less serious cases, may be content to reprimand or warn; but it must respect the individual's freedom of behaviour and not invade his personality. The man for whom the ordinary suspended sentence was conceived was that 'rational man who is master of himself' in the Declaration of Rights, 1789, and the free contractant of the Napoleonic Code, 1804.

(Ancel 1971: 37)

Though in the civil (or statute) law tradition of much of continental Europe the element of suspension was also fundamental, the suspension (or *sursis* – literally postponement) was of the execution not imposition of sentence. Because it was conditional on good behaviour the *sursis* is sometimes referred to as a *conditional sentence*; to those familiar with the Anglo-Saxon system it is more recognizable as a suspended sentence, though not necessarily of prison.

The essential features of conditional sentence were:

- *pronouncement of sentence*,
- the decision that *execution of sentence will be suspended*, providing that the convicted person does not commit another offence or crime punished by a prison sentence during the probation period,
- revocation of suspension of sentence in the event of a relapse,
- the consideration that the *sentence did not occur* if the offender has fulfilled his obligations.[6] (Cartledge *et al.* 1981: 20).

In its original Belgian and French form (in the *loi Lejeune* of 1888 and the *loi Bérenger* of 1891 respectively) the *sursis* was a trial period between imposition and execution of sentence. Its central tenet was not, as was the case in most common law countries, the provision of advice and guidance, but the suspension itself. Both the *loi Lejeune* and the *loi Bérenger* provided for the suspension of fines or imprisonment in the case of defendants not previously imprisoned, with the sentence activated automatically in the event of a further serious offence during the suspension. Probation therefore must be distinguished from supervision:[7] it is the suspension not the supervision which constitutes probation:

in England and Massachusetts, probation developed specifically with a view to the reclamation of offenders. ... The primary purpose of the introduction of statutory provision for the conditional suspension of punishment on the Continent was to provide a *suitable alternative to short-term imprisonment*, and to avoid the contamination of juvenile, first, and petty offenders in prison.

(United Nations 1951: 203–4; emphasis in original)

Hence the comment of the originator of the Belgian *sursis*, Jules Lejeune, during the debate on its proposed introduction in the House of Representatives in 1888:

Those for the benefit of whom the conditional sentence has been created, have no need of the assistance of protective supervision (*patronage*). They will reform by themselves.

(cited in United Nations 1951: 64)

Many European criminal codes, influenced by the French Revolution, reflected a concern to ensure that a sentence was imposed in respect of a crime (an acknowledgement of the necessity of maintaining the rule of law) and to legislate against the abuse of state power by maximizing the objectivity of sentencing arrangements. In a legal context in which even traditional acts of clemency such as admonition by a judge were perceived as threats to the rights of man, to involve an executive expert in the administration of justice and the determination of sentence on extra-judicial grounds would be unacceptable.

In France the Revolution marked an abrupt change from complex and arbitrary systems of justice such as the *lettres de cachet* which appertained under the *ancien régime* where the King was above the law. The Constituent Assembly introduced a principle of strict legality into the Penal Codes of 1791 and 1810 in the belief that the criminal code could not be too precise (Ancel 1971: 5, 21), creating what Radzinowicz has called 'the iron equation of crime and punishment affirmed by the classical codes' (in Ancel 1971: vii) and making the judge a mere dispenser of punishment (see Wills 1981).

By the late nineteenth century the ambition of basing the justice system on principles of strict commensurability or proportionality (terms defined and distinguished by Walker 1985: 108) was mediated by several factors:

- a disillusionment with prisons. Prisons had not been used for punishment under the *ancien régime*, and confidence in their reformist (or even prophylactic) potential had been shaken by increased recidivism and an increasingly dominant perception of their contaminating potential;
- scepticism as to the sufficiency of commensurability or proportionality as a basis for the penal code. Adherence to classical justice (relating the punishment to the crime not the character or previous behaviour of the criminal) mediated against mercy in the cases of minor or first offenders and those who evoked human sympathy, and in the light of this attempts had been made in different countries from the early nineteenth century to reinstate such merciful disposals as judicial admonition. Classical justice, however, militated against toughness as well as mercy and there was at this time increasing political embarrassment at the proliferation of recidivists. The promise of greater punishment for such people was influential in gaining acceptance of flexibility, and the full title of the *loi Bérenger* was 'on the progressive augmentation of sentences in the case of recidivism and on their mitigation for first offences';
- this discussion was of jurisprudential importance across much of continental Europe:

  A new conception of punishment was born: from being a means of expiation for the fault committed, punishment had to become an effective instrument for the improvement of the offender, which led logically to the question of *alternative sentences*.

  (Ancel 1971: 8)

- scepticism about classical justice was related to positive criminology's increasingly influential perception of crime as curable disease. Such was the influence of this line of thought on the administration of justice that there emerged a discourse in which post-Darwinian scientific logic came close to *replacing* the judicial logic of classical criminology in the determination of sentence – a substitution seen by some as actually enhancing individual liberty by the scientific application of 'cure':

  The sentence was no longer thought of as a modern version of the ancient practice of branding the criminal with a red-hot iron: it was applied to an individual according to his personal characteristics, assessed biologically, psychologically and anthropologically.

(Ancel 1971: 10)

- as a result of a growing internationalism in criminology and criminal justice, information became available about experiments with suspensive sentences in Austria, Germany, Italy, Portugal, Russia and Switzerland. This internationalism disseminated and legitimated departures from nation-state sentencing traditions, and many countries were debating or introducing proposals to replace execution of sentence with admonition or suspension. Hence the *sursis* was debated at the International Association for Penal Law in Brussels in 1889 and at International Penitentiary Conferences in Rome in 1885, St Petersburg in 1890 and Paris in 1895, with proponents supporting the minimization of sentence in trivial cases and opponents arguing that conditional sentences were wrong in principle and would open the door to arbitrariness and oppression (Ancel 1971: 9). It was at the Paris Conference that a resolution expressing approval of the *sursis* was adopted (United Nations 1951: 65–6).

The Franco-Belgian system spread rapidly, being adopted in Luxembourg, Portugal, Norway, the Netherlands, Bulgaria, Italy, Sweden, Spain, Hungary, Greece, Finland and the Swiss cantons of Geneva, Vaud, Wallis, Tessin, Fribourg, Neuchâtel, Basle Town, Basle Land, Lucerne and Schaffhausen. The systems remained varied (Grünhut 1948: 298), being designed to solve local problems in a manner consonant with the local character and politics of criminal justice. In all cases, however, suspension was a privilege not a right, and not available for partial implementation, the idea of a 'mixed' sentence being introduced much later.[8]

Originally the sursis was:

- as much an institution of law as the fine or prison, with execution suspended only when particular criteria had been met, in circumstances approved by statute and at the behest of a judge whose discretion was firmly guided. Any notion of suspending the *imposition* of sentence would have been unacceptable: *the sursis* was imposed within a jurisprudential framework which decreed that to fail to punish was an abuse of power. A further offence normally led to the *sursis* being nulled, and to the execution of sentence without a further court appearance;

- not, as with the common law tradition, a framework into which additional conditions could be fitted, for it was deemed wrong in principle for an offender on *sursis* to be subject to requirements additional to the law. Though details differed, to comply with the injunction not to commit a further offence led to retrospective erasure of the penalty. While voluntary welfare organizations, often connected with the Church, may have been used to support vulnerable offenders, and arrangements for the supervision of juveniles were predicated on a different basis, to make a requirement with sanctions attached to non-compliance would have been an unacceptable intrusion:

> It is not a question of bad behaviour or of what is called, in a system of supervised freedom, an 'incident'; only a legally defined offence can bring the offender back before the penal judge.
>
> (Ancel 1971: 36)

The years following World War One saw the augmentation of suspension by supervision across much of Western Europe as professional expertise, described by Radzinowicz as the conditional sentence's 'more adventurous and adaptable sister' (Ancel 1971: vii), gained acceptability. Accordingly *sursis surveillée*, or *sursis avec mise à l'épreuve*, began to emerge as additional sentencing options to *sursis simple*. At this point a conflation of 'probation' with 'supervision' occurred in the majority of western countries, which at differing speeds began to move towards the acceptance of extra-legal variables in sentencing:

> The common law procedure with its interval between two distinct decisions – conviction and sentence – facilitated a suspension of the promulgation of a sentence, and the abstention from even a hypothetical punishment strengthens the rehabilitative forces of probation. Courts were not restricted in the use of probation by statutory limitations. Supervision became indispensable and took more and more the form of professional casework by trained social workers of the court. The *sursis*, however, never lost its character of a particular act of leniency, granted to offenders who deserved it in exceptional circumstances. Legislation, therefore, provided guarantees against abuse by unwarranted application of this measure.
>
> (United Nations 1959: 3)

The process occurred only gradually across continental Europe, however:

- in **Austria** the *sursis* was introduced in 1920 but without an adult supervisory system until a trial period in 1966. Supervised probation became permanent in 1980 when, in a break with the *sursis* tradition, special provision was enacted for drug offenders, whose proceedings could be halted in return for their acceptance of supervision for two years (Cartledge *et al.* 1981: 42);
- in **Belgium**, though the *loi Lejeune* of 1888 empowered courts to impose a suspended sentence, only in 1948 was it acknowledged that supervision would extend the utility of the *sursis* to those unable to reform unaided. A draft Probation Bill was discussed in the 1950s but the modern probation system was only introduced in 1964;
- in **Denmark**, one of the first countries to introduce supervision (by volunteer charitable organizations) as a facility in 1905 as part of a system of conditional sentence (United Nations 1954a: 144; United Nations 1954b: 38), the *sursis* was a major part of the criminal justice system almost since its initiation, though as late as the 1950s only half the *sursis* imposed were *sursis surveillées*. Not until 1973 was responsibility for probation transferred to the Ministry of Justice (*Justitsministeren*), so merging the activities of the Danish Welfare Association with those of the Prison Administration;
- in **France**, in spite of the *loi Bérenger* of 1891, experiments with adult probation only occurred in the early 1950s, when some *tribunaux correctionels*[9] began to use it within the existing legal framework. Attempts were then made to draft a statute to adapt probation to French law so as to address concerns about probation's judicial propriety. These led to the introduction of an adult probation system in 1958, le *milieu ouvert* (Code of Criminal Procedure 1957) on the basis of *le sursis avec le mis à l'épreuve*;
- in **Germany** no adult probation system existed before World War Two, though a power of discontinuance akin to a conditional pardon (*bedingte Begnadigung*) was available to the Ministry of Justice from 1895 until its abandonment by the National Socialists in 1943 as incompatible with the authority of the state (United Nations 1951: 67–9). After the war the

Bundestag's interest in the English system, particularly in relation to juveniles, led to a meeting in 1950 at Bad Godesberg between German representatives and staff of the British Home Office. The result was a probation plan, drawn up by two senior judges, Lingemann and Clostermann, proposing supervision accompanied by a suspension of the imposition of sentence. This was operational in five courts in the Federal Republic by 1951 (Grünhut 1952: 171). Federal legislation for supervision by trained officers was introduced in 1953 for juveniles and 1954 for adults with each *land* responsible for the employment of its officers and the organization of its service;

- in **Switzerland** probation normally without supervision (*Schutzaufsicht*) was introduced by cantonal legislation, and existed in ten of the twenty-five cantons by the mid-1920s. The Federal Penal Code of 1937 required provision for an adult *sursis simple* to exist in all cantons by this year and for a *sursis surveillée* in 1942, though acceptance of the system was slow through the widespread belief that the *sursis* was a 'let-off'.

Though in much of continental Europe probation's origins differ from the common law tradition, almost from the first common law exerted influence on developments there, and continental countries themselves were variably enthusiastic in their embrace of the *sursis*:

- in **Belgium** in a departure from the strict principle of the *sursis* the Probation Law of 1964 provided for the postponement of sentencing, at the request of the defendant and in very restricted circumstances, for between one and five years:

  > It had long been felt that legislation which would allow imprisonment and its injurious consequences to be obviated in carefully chosen cases was needed in Belgium. The idea of such legislation was unquestionably inspired by the experiments carried out in the Anglo-Saxon countries.
  >
  > (Council of Europe 1970: 92)

- in **Denmark** conditional sentences exist alongside the Anglo-Saxon system; conditions such as restrictions on alcohol or drug use, treatment requirements and regulations as to how financial commitments are to be met may be added to the sentence;
- in **Finland** though probation for minors and adults, introduced in 1918, was again based on the *sursis*, from the first super-

visors had enforcement powers unacceptable under the Franco-Belgian system: revocation was possible should probationers fall into habits of 'intemperance, viciousness, or a depraved life' (Trought 1927: 73), fail to keep the supervisor informed of their place of residence and work, leave either without permission or return having been removed by the supervisor (United Nations 1954a);

- in **France** the 1958 system of *sursis avec le mis à l'épreuve* was 'based on the probation system of the English-speaking countries' (Council of Europe 1970: 118) involving supervision, support and the enforcement of specific obligations. It could be 'mixed' with a fine and was nullified on successful completion;

- in the **Netherlands** the influence of the *sursis* was modulated by the country's strong historical and cultural links with Britain, the involvement of Church-related organizations (the Salvation Army Probation Department, Catholic–Protestant Association, Protestant Christian Probation Association, Roman Catholic Rehabilitation Society and Dr F.S. Meijer Association for disturbed adolescents) (van Swaaningen and uit Beijerse 1993) and a fairly relaxed perception of the relation between state and citizen. Suspending sentences of less than a year was permitted as early as 1915, with conditions, such as supervision on a 'free patron system' which involved supporting and guiding discharged prisoners as well as fighting for penal reform (Heijder 1967), being permissible attachments to the suspension. Most restrictions on the use of conditional sentences were removed in 1951 on the principle that:

> enforcement of a penalty must also give an opportunity of facilitating the social rehabilitation of the prisoner. Under this principle, an approach to penal matters is being developed in which greater account is taken of the individual situation of each prisoner and in which collaboration with the probation institute will take a new form and content – even during imprisonment. ... The result of this has been not only that the number of delinquents dealt with by probation institutions has risen, but also that there has been an increasing tendency to leave it to probation institutions to carry out treatment.
>
> (Council of Europe 1970: 187–8)

Though probation (*reclassering*) is now a professionalized social work activity with statutory functions, like Austria but unlike the Scandinavian countries where the trend has been for voluntary probation organizations to be taken over by the state, many officers are still employed by voluntary organizations. They continue to be influential apologists for a tolerant penal policy in a country where liberal values are hegemonic (Downes 1982; 1988) in spite of the fact that the organizations' financial dependence on the Ministry of Justice has diminished their traditional autonomy (Woelinga 1990);

- in **Sweden** a probation law was promulgated in 1918 based on the *sursis* but with supervision by policemen, members of a prisoners' aid society or volunteers from the professions, trade or commerce, involving 'general *watchfulness*, and assistance to the offender in living a law-abiding life' (United Nations 1951: 153). Since 1942 provision has existed for suspending the imposition of sentence, probation constituting a gateway to therapy and control, with permissible conditions of orders including abstention from alcohol, submission to hospital treatment (for alcoholism or other purposes), submission to restrictions on the use of earnings and restitution for losses occasioned by the offence.

Whereas in common law countries from informal and marginal beginnings probation became a dimension of law and policy, in civil law countries supervision was grafted on to a *sursis* whose main function was not to influence and support but to suspend the execution of a sentence subject to good behaviour. While in Britain probation without supervision would be incomprehensible (the two words are frequently used interchangeably), under civil law such a separation was both common and necessary: suspension was basic, supervision a later accretion.

PROBATION AFTER WORLD WAR TWO

If I were asked which, among the modern methods for the treatment of offenders is the most promising, without hesitation I would say: probation. ... If every country had an adequate system of probation the immediate result would be an automatic reduction of the prison population and consequently of the number of prisons.

(López-Rey 1957: 346)

If community programmes were *replacing* institutions, then systems high in community places would show a less than average use of institutions. But if community was *supplementing* institutions, then systems high in community would also have an above-average use of institutions and this is just what seems to be happening.

(Cohen 1985: 49)

Probation received renewed international attention following World War Two. In Britain the London Probation Service was developing international links with Canada, West Germany and the Netherlands and such was the overseas interest in the probation and juvenile court systems that the British Council brought students for training from France, Italy, Spain, Greece, the Lebanon, Uruguay and Singapore (Page 1992: 224–5).

The period also saw a number of initiatives undertaken by the United Nations. The Social Commission of the Economic and Social Council included probation as a priority subject in its work programme on the prevention of crime and the treatment of offenders, commissioning and publishing a major cross-national study of some 400 pages and containing 284 references, entitled *Probation and Related Measures* (United Nations 1951; see also López-Rey 1957; 1976). In 1950, on the basis of advice from the Secretary-General's International Group of Experts on the Prevention of Crime and the Treatment of Offenders, the UN Council supported a programme of study and research to complement *Probation and Related Measures*. This led first to a major European seminar on probation, held in London at the invitation of HM Government in 1952, its proceedings being published two years later (United Nations 1954a), and secondly to a further study, prepared by Max Grünhut of Oxford University (United Nations 1954b).

By this time the dominance of positivist explanations of criminality seemed unassailable, , with probation supervision perceived as a logical and progressive, indeed necessary, disposal. The 1952 seminar brought together twelve experts, fifty-eight delegates from seventeen European countries comprising representatives of the judiciary, correctional administration, social work training and social welfare administration (United Nations 1954a: vi) and observers from twenty-four organizations. Delegates were confident in their embrace of clinical techniques and their belief in probation's potential (United Nations 1954a: 1; for a similar picture from a British government source see Home Office 1956).

Parts of the seminar were experiential in presentation. Delegates saw a government film, *Probation Officer*, and witnessed a dramatized presentation of the work of the probation officer in court.[10] In striking contrast to the civil law ethos, the spirit and method of supervision, 'the process of helping the offender to re-establish himself in society by means of positive treatment in the open', was deemed more important than administrative and legal considerations, and 'surveillance as such took second place to effective help given by the probation officer to the person in his care'. Probation was a social treatment which should be free of 'limitations of a general and mandatory nature', and selection of probationers should be based on scientific, including where necessary medico-psychological, examination (United Nations 1954a: 1–4).

To delegates, conditions imposed by magistrates should be sufficiently flexible to leave the probation officer room for manoeuvre because of the service's professionalism: 'The era which relied solely on charity, goodwill and simple personal intuition' was long past, and use should be made of volunteers only for financial reasons or because their 'enthusiasm might serve as a safeguard against administrative routine'. Officers should be of 'good intelligence, emotional maturity, good health, and a satisfactory general and professional education'; training should concentrate on psychological and psychiatric problems and comprise both a general grounding taken jointly with other social service workers and a specialized study of casework as applied to delinquents (United Nations 1954a: 6–7).

Both the speed and extent of the shift from classicism in the continental European jurisdictions will be evident, as will the confidence with which different probation services assumed an unequivocally professional *persona*, spurning the idea that their tools were integrity, commonsense and experience of the world, and restricting almost with contempt the contribution of volunteers. The therapeutic self-confidence of this conference represents the apotheosis of clinical probation work. Using circular logic it applied to its own activities the interpretations it used to understand crime and criminals: clinical methods declared clinical methods triumphant. Basing its self-evaluation on experience and wisdom rather than effectiveness data of the kind which were to contribute to the downfall of the perspective a generation later, 1950s probation produced an unanswerable self-justification: if its work defied empirical verification the fault lay not with the clinical paradigm but with the tools of measurement.

The study *Practical Results and Financial Aspects of Adult Probation in Selected Countries* (United Nations 1954b), having given accounts of adult probation in twelve jurisdictions notes both difference and commonality: differences related primarily to administration, the place of probation in different legal systems and the use of volunteers, but common ground existed in the expansion of the system to embrace adults:

> Everywhere, adult probation has passed the stage where it was regarded, almost with suspicion, as some further measure of exceptional leniency, or accepted only as a mere substitute for undesirable short prison sentences. Adult probation has come into its own and has been acknowledged, at least in principle, as a constructive method of treatment, indispensable, beside prison and other forms of institutional care, in any system aiming at individual prevention of criminality.
>
> (United Nations 1954b: 79)

In 1954 the UN Social Commission requested a further study of probation, including selection (United Nations 1959). The study reflects again Grünhut's enthusiastic endorsement of probation, which with juvenile courts he regarded as the greatest advance of twentieth-century penology, a measure which, while it could potentially be used with scientific precision, also provided an opportunity to take responsible risks in humanitarian interests:

> those responsible for the selection of offenders for probation look for positive assets in the offender's life which make probation possible, and for faults and defects which make probation necessary. In the final judgement, a balance must be made between the two opposing forces, and the decisive question is whether probation can be made use of to put and keep this person's life on the right track. If there are positive assets only there appears to be no need for probation, and the court may resort to conditional discharge or a fine. Where the negative factors are too strong, a more intense form of treatment will be necessary.
>
> (United Nations 1959: 18)

Since the 1960s and 1970s probation has in many countries become increasingly systematized. In Australia, Canada, Britain and New Zealand it has come to be identified as an appropriate strategy of control for adults, while in the traditionally punitive criminal justice system of the United States it has acquired a strong correctional orientation but without central organization. In parts of continental Europe somewhat similar developments have occurred. For example:

- in **Finland**, where responsibility for probation was assumed by the Probation and After-Care Association (*Kriminaalihuoltoyhdistys*) in 1975, and where there are currently some 260 full-time probation officers, all with a higher degree in social or behavioural sciences or a first degree in social work, both the probation system and legislation governing it are in transition. The work of the *Kriminaalihuoltoyhdistys* is moving in the direction of implementing community sanctions as alternatives to the traditionally high incarceration rate, and a community service system encompassing the entire country was introduced in April 1994;
- in **Germany** enhanced or intensive probation was introduced for higher risk offenders in 1975; this involves being placed under a particular supervising centre (*Aufsichtstelle*) and probation officer who work together to ensure effective control and public protection (Cartledge *et al.* 1981: 136);
- in **Sweden** probation was integrated with the correctional system in 1964; in 1965 a new Penal Code introduced non-institutional care as probation (*skyddstillsyn*), a sanction in its own right (Cartledge *et al.* 1981: 408). Following a further process of integration with the prison system in 1992, probation is administered in fifty-four districts under the Ministry of Justice, and accountable to national and local Supervision Boards responsible for managing supervision itself.

Today probation in much of the world is addressing the problem of how to deal firmly with offenders and still reduce the prison population. Probation in this sense constitutes one of the clearest future 'visions' of social control. This vision is characterized by the twin processes of convergence and diversification: convergence as two systems become a heterogeneous whole, and diversification as probation moves away from a unified 'casework' approach into activities which include supervising community service, reparation schemes, community corrections and brokerage – hiring and monitoring private sector agencies brought in to supervise and control.

TWO INFLUENCES ON THE DEVELOPMENT OF PROBATION

Two influences are particularly relevant to the development of probation, and the conflation of the common and civil law traditions: the juvenile court movement and positivist criminology. We say something of each in turn.

Juvenile justice

Though our concern is primarily with adult jurisdictions it is through the juvenile justice system that a loosening of the statutory basis of continental probation has often been effected. The acceptance of probation supervision in relation to juveniles has contributed to a climate in which the imposition of similar requirements on adults has been more acceptable; indeed in countries such as Malaysia, where probation remains at an early stage of development, it continues to exist as a social welfare facility solely for juveniles.

Though supervisory probation typically spread in common law countries through colonial influence, the existence of a nonconformist temperance tradition and the early and effective organization of a probation lobby, it was in respect of juveniles that its diversification from inebriate or first offenders usually began. Children were generally perceived as immature, and they almost invariably had less than full citizenship rights. In the late nineteenth century they were the subjects of political interest in the United States as well as Britain (Platt 1969). In Britain the control of families over their children was being undermined by the state: Education Acts of 1870, 1891 and 1897 defined elementary education as a state responsibility, the first child protection legislation was introduced in the 1870s (Parton 1985), and the notion of the 'child as citizen' emphasized a direct link between state and child, by-passing the father as intermediate between the two and repudiating any implication that the child was the father's property.

Children became ideal recipients of compulsory reformation,

and probation supervision a third front to be summoned in when family and school had failed. It offered an amalgam of care and control akin to good child rearing practice, and the changing social and political status of children, explored more fully elsewhere (Harris 1995; Harris and Timms 1993a), is hence of real if indirect relevance to our current study.

Civil law countries which by reference to the rights of man upheld the necessity of statute law against the oppressive potential of executive decision-making proved less solicitous of the rights of children, more inclined to define the proper social response to juvenile delinquency in educational terms, and so more willing to respond paternalistically to their perceived needs and interests. Accordingly, in civil as well as common law jurisdictions juvenile supervision became a means of socializing the deviant young which circumvented the objections of jurists to adult probation. These objections took a number of forms:

- the impropriety of a decision to 'not sentence' a known offender, given the obligation placed upon societies by some classical jurists to exact retribution (for a convenient discussion of this Kantian categorical obligation see Honderich 1969: Chapter 2). With juveniles, however, most countries had a tradition of greater flexibility and tolerance whether or not it was fully reflected in statute law. Supervising a child was therefore a comprehensible extension of the control traditionally exercised over children by family, church, school or apprentice master;

- the transfer of *de facto* responsibility from the judiciary to the executive. That unsentenced offenders could be dealt with on the basis not (or not only) of an offence but of operational decisions taken by professionals based on their view of the offenders' response to probation thus far raised constitutional objections from classical jurists; but these objections lost much force in respect of children once it became possible to define delinquency in terms of educational or welfare deficit. This definition legitimated precisely the modes of supervision so unacceptable in respect of adult offenders;

- the departure from the tenets of classical justice involved in individualized sentencing. As we have seen, supervised probation was individualized at the point of *disposition* because the disposal was normally less severe than would be considered appropriate, and in its *exercise*. Though in some jurisdictions

minimum contact requirements exist we have nowhere found a statement of acceptable maxima, or even of strong norms of reporting frequency, duration or content; and it seems, in the politico-legal context of the time, a prerequisite for the exercise of individualized justice for its objects to have less than full citizenship status – a requirement met perfectly by children;
• the enforcement by executive action of behavioural requirements which included restrictions on living and working arrangements – areas in which absolute freedom was fundamental to non-totalitarian societies – was perceived as having repressive potential in respect of adults. It was, however, almost universally accepted as a necessary aspect of child rearing, for all developed societies impose restrictions on the personal, social and sexual behaviour of children which do not exist in respect of adults.

Certainly the early predominance of juveniles in probation work in both civil and common law countries is noticeable:

• in **Australia**, where strong cultural objections to the spread of adult probation existed, it became the favoured disposal for juveniles following World War One, being exercised by three categories of staff: stipendiary probation officers (in Victoria, Western Australia and Tasmania), officials of Child Welfare or Public Relief Departments (in New South Wales, Queensland and South Australia) and voluntary probation officers (United Nations 1951: 54);
• in **Belgium**, home of the original *sursis*, supervision (*liberté surveillée*) was introduced in the Child Protection Law 1912, with supervision by volunteer *délégués à la protection de l'enfance* (Trought 1927; United Nations 1954a). In 1946 a number of public prosecutors (*parquets*), taking the lead from the *parquet* of Ghent, made experimental use of probation in selected juvenile cases, charges being allowed to lapse in the event of good conduct. This experiment came to be known as Praetorian probation;
• in **Denmark**, from 1922 each municipality was required to have an elected Child Welfare (or Protective) Council (*Vägeraad*) to determine the supervision or out-of-home placement of children; at this time any citizen under the age of 60 could by law be called on to supervise a child as a *délégué* (Trought 1927: 53).

In some areas the *Vägeraad* performed the role of court as well as executive agency;

- in **France** arrangements for *liberté surveillée* were introduced in the Juvenile Court Law 1912, with supervision by volunteer members of welfare societies. By 1924, at least in Paris, investigations were made by a field worker required to report on the child's character and environment, and supervision was the responsibility of a *délégué à la liberté surveillée*, the 'delegate' of the judge appointed to supervise delinquents, normally a member of a charitable organization or legal defence committee (Trought 1927: 82–4);
- in **Germany** before the Third Reich each *land* had a juvenile probation system. The protective supervision (*schutzaufsicht*) introduced under the Youth Welfare Act 1922 was mainly undertaken by volunteer welfare workers, though with a small number of supervisors paid by the *land*, municipality, district or commune.

As late as the 1950s even though the immediate post-war tendency in high crime areas was to cope with an increase in juvenile crime by greater use of the fine at the expense of probation (Grünhut 1956: 74–5), juvenile offenders comprised 75 per cent of all probationers in Britain. Though some countries had more people on probation than in prison this was so only when juveniles and adults were aggregated: in Britain the numbers of adult probationers comprised less than 74 per cent of the adult prison population, and when men alone were included the proportion dropped to 54 per cent (United Nations 1954b: 80).

Positivist criminology

The second significant feature in the spread and legitimation of probation was positivist criminology, whose effective origins are normally associated with the publication in 1876 of Lombroso's *L'Uomo Delinquente* (for a useful and accessible discussion see Taylor *et al*. 1973: Chapters 1–2). In its radical form positivism offered a new paradigm for comprehending crime which gave legitimacy to probation as a social and psychological intervention. If classical jurists were to accept any departure from the tenets of justice, however, any new paradigm would have to meet two conditions:

- to justify the need for change it would have to mount an effective challenge to the legitimacy of the existing framework;
- it would have to promise alternative but immutable aetiological laws and rules of conduct in a form no less coherent than that which it replaced.

A biological framework which classified crime as a curable phenomenon could meet both these criteria. First the paradigm shift which involved regarding the offender as other-than-rational or other-than-free repudiated as unjust in its own terms a sentencing framework which addressed the crime not the criminal. Second, in a climate of cynicism at the failure of existing systems to stem a perceived increase in criminal activity across much of Western Europe, positivism offered a possibility of cure. Though the influence of radical positivism was to be patchy and short lived, inserting a medical element into conventional understandings of criminal justice paved the way for the twentieth-century psychiatrization of crime, and for the confidence expressed by the correctional experts at the United Nations European probation seminar (United Nations 1954a).

In Britain the introduction of probation reflected increasing dissatisfaction with the 'uniform treatment' theories of nineteenth-century penology, whose damaging consequences[11] in the prisons contrasted with the optimism inspired by the police court missionaries. The influence of European positivism in Britain was always modulated by a robust scepticism and desire for administrative efficiency, and supposedly scientific uniform penalties were increasingly attracting public opprobrium for failing to reform or deter numerous minor offenders.

For example, two-thirds of women prisoners had been committed for drunkenness, which was regarded as being as closely associated with prostitution as female drug dependence is today (Priestley 1985: 72), and presented problems which the system had failed to address (Forsythe 1987; 1993). In relation to children, in spite of the rapid development of reformatory schools (Carpenter 1851) children of less than 12 were being committed to prison for crimes such as larceny; until 1899 reformatory school disposals were used in addition to not instead of hard labour; and in spite of the increased attention being given to juvenile offenders many were in practice receiving treatment similar to that afforded recidivists (see Rose 1967: Chapter 1).

As the century advanced, influenced not only by continental European positivism but Christian reformism, and under pressure from the pragmatic character of the British administrative tradition (see Thomas 1972), differentiation and individualism took over from uniformity as governing principles of penal policy. Differentiation embraced first children, conceiving them as immature beings particularly amenable to influence for good or ill, and the insane, extending to young adults and female offenders by the end of the century.

This equivocal move towards differentiation is epitomized in the Gladstone Report (Report from the Departmental Committee on Prisons 1895) which, influenced by the reformist discourse, argued that crime should be set in a social context with attention given to reformation as well as punishment. Gladstone accordingly argued for improvements in prison conditions, the abolition of unproductive labour, the extension of prison libraries, restrictions on flogging and the encouragement of visiting preachers to augment the efforts of prison chaplains.

In addition, and crucially for the development of probation, the Report turned its attention to the experiences of prisoners on release. Though it would be incorrect to believe this was a new concern, Gladstone marked a shift in emphasis from the threatening to the reformist, and the treatment of young offenders in particular was seen as the key to future prevention; the Probation of Offenders Act 1907 put the probation service on a statutory footing;[12] recognition of training Borstals came with the Prevention of Crime Act 1908; the Mental Deficiency Act 1913 aimed, following Gladstone's recommendations, to rid the prisons of feeble-minded recidivists; and the Criminal Justice Administration Act 1914 sought, by introducing the 'time to pay' principle into fine administration, to reduce the frequency of imprisonment for default. In short, probation was one part of a broader set of changes in penal policy

In Britain, therefore, the origins of probation are best regarded less as an outpouring of positivist confidence than as a response to disillusionment with the pre-psychological positivism which appertained in the prisons. The outcome of debates predicated on the belief that prisons were human laboratories and prisoners variables for manipulation had proved neither empirically encouraging nor culturally acceptable. The shift to probation reflected a belief in the exercise of influence based on wise advice, good example and

care and control of the kind to be found in the good family of which
so many criminals had demonstrably been deprived. The 'human
laboratory' argument was now widely discredited:

> While scientific and more particularly medical observation and
> experience are of the most essential value in guiding opinion
> on the whole subject, it would be a loss of time to search for
> a perfect system in learned but conflicting theories, when so
> much can be done by the recognition of the plain fact that the
> great majority of prisoners are ordinary men and women
> amenable, more or less, to all those influences which affect
> persons outside.
>
> (Report from the Departmental Committee on Prisons 1895)

In the United States the impact of European positivism on penal
theory was greater than in Britain, primarily as a result of the
hegemonic influence of the medical profession on contemporary
explanations of human behaviour. Culturally as well as politically
there is in the United States a strong interest in the constitutional
dimensions of human behaviour (Wilson and Herrnstein 1985). In
relation to crime causation, however, such notions intersect with
an equally strong puritanism to create an explanatory awkwardness characteristic of much American criminology today. In the
nineteenth century positivism had combined with a theologically
induced perception of offenders as morally inferior beings to
create a model of the atavistic criminal. This led to a justification
of prison 'medical' experiments and to a discourse which used
criminal anthropology, heredity and feeble-mindedness as contrib-
utors to an aetiology of crime, a discourse which in turn was a
precursor of the early twentieth-century interest in eugenics,
taught in three-quarters of American universities in the years
following World War One (Karmen 1980: 89–90):

> Theories of crime causation in the nineteenth century did not
> develop in isolation or in a vacuum. Their cultural setting
> included advancements in biology, in medicine, in psychiatry,
> in psychology and in sociology. In these disciplines were found
> the scientific or quasi-scientific explanations of man, his body,
> his mind, his actions, his society. It was inevitable that man's
> behavior – especially his criminal behavior – should come
> within the province of specialists in these fields.
>
> (Fink 1938: 240)

Probation's confident post-war assumption of a therapeutic orientation downgraded the importance of the offence in comparison with the therapeutic potential of the offender and did little to grapple with the relation between probation as a gesture of help and the legal question of whether a 'guilty mind' existed. If the offender was rational the clemency implicit in probation supervision might appear unjustifiable; if not, not only was the legitimacy of the criminal justice system as a whole called into question but probation was seemingly operating within the wrong paradigm.

Though on a workaday basis this contradiction was normally contained by reference to concepts such as 'pressure', 'crisis', 'acting out of character' and 'compassion' – concepts as much moral as clinical (for such, perhaps, is the reality if not the theory of much clinical work of this kind), on occasion an awkwardness became manifest. For example, part of the purpose of the Criminal Justice Act 1948 was to extend the use of probation for mentally disordered offenders by means of a treatment requirement of up to one year. Yet while this statutory restriction on the length of treatment time reflected a concern with civil rights more than clinical diagnosis (Grünhut 1963: 48), what would happen if, the order having been made, a psychiatrist stated that treatment would not be efficacious and chose to discharge the probationer from hospital?

This kind of problem has subsequently been addressed by probation assuming a more precise sentencing location. In Britain this began in the late 1960s with an expansion in size and responsibility, and with the beginning of the discussion as to the possibility of probation becoming central to a community correctional strategy located at the centre of the penal stage (Haxby 1978; see also Faulkner 1989). As we have seen, however, this line of argument, which culminated in the transformation of probation into a sentence in its own right, necessitates a revision of probation's values and orientation. Further, when set alongside the opposite move in the civil law countries towards greater flexibility and professional autonomy it has so blurred the distinctions between the civil and common law traditions as to render them meaningless.

CONCLUSION

> The assets of criminal law as the most advanced institution of 'formal social control' include impartiality, objectivity and equality. But these assets are counterbalanced by a liability, namely the stark inability of positive criminal law to restore the social equilibrium or balance that has been disturbed by an event which has been defined as criminal.
>
> (Pelikan 1991: 159)

> Sometimes the legally ignorant common sense of the colonists brought about improvements in criminal justice. Sometimes also it led to peculiarly American institutions which have left their mark upon our legal system.
>
> (Pound 1975: 82)

Though probation raises contrasting issues in the common and civil law traditions neither is homogeneous, and it would be incorrect to assume that after the initial impetus developments were driven by system origin. Material factors (notably the availability of resources), political considerations (including a reluctance to be over-kind to offenders), organizational realities (the sophistication and responsiveness of local administrative structures), cultural norms and geography have all influenced developments. Though Old Commonwealth countries imported probation from Britain, the import was quickly overlain by features which gave Australian, Canadian and Indian probation their own character; while in the United States the common law approach of Massachusetts proved by no means typical and the diversity of American probation today is such as to render dubious even the use of the word 'system' to describe it.

Developmentally certain distinctions exist between common and civil law countries, even though much convergence has now occurred. In the common law tradition development has been from the relatively unfettered discretion of judges to impose probation-as-mercy or probation-as-therapy for minor offenders to a recognition of probation as a personal intrusion, an investment of resources and a dimension of penal policy. In the civil law tradition development has entailed addressing a principled objection to discretionary sentences by substituting a paradigm of scientific positivism for classical justice and acknowledging the advantages of permitting experts to respond to changes in attitude, behaviour or circumstance as they occur. Ironically, probation's development in some civil law jurisdictions was also aided by the political inconvenience of the impossibility under classical justice of sentencing recidivists up as well as sentencing minor offenders down (Ancel 1971).

From quite early in the history of probation it was becoming clear that its common law basis was liable to be changed once it was exported to the Empire. Equally in the United States the importance of the Constitution and the relative autonomy of states, counties, towns and districts so far as operational probation was concerned created variations in practice, and conflict between Supreme Court interpretations of the Constitution and the common law tradition. As Roscoe Pound noted in his Harvard lectures of 1923:

> The cleavage between common law and legislation, which runs through every department, is a characteristic feature of our law. The American lawyer must keep in mind two sets of rules, traditional or common law on the one hand, and statutory on the other. ... The traditional or common law potentially covers the whole field but is superseded at numerous points by detailed statutory rules, or even by complete statutory provisions for some one subject, or in some particular field.
>
> (Pound 1975: 142)

Historically these conflicts related to the powers of courts in relation to suspension (see Chute and Bell 1956: 67–71 for a discussion of the debates in Vermont and Missouri in particular) and the constitutional rights which accrued to offenders by dint of the *existence* of probation (that in particular circumstances the possibility of making a probation order must be considered prior to sentence being passed) or of *being on* probation (that though there is no right to probation, once given it cannot be revoked without a court hearing) (Hink 1962).

In Canada and Australia there was neither the political will nor the administrative capacity to develop a coherent system. In vast, sparsely populated terrains supervision was seldom practical, a lack of enthusiasm for caring for offenders was manifest and probation attracted little attention until after World War Two. Whereas much of post-war Europe embraced a practice based on positivist criminology in which the therapeutic function of probation was a necessary corrective to legalism, in the colonies the discourse was robustly individualistic, with probation coming into its own only when, through association with community sanctions, it found a more culturally consonant niche.

In India we see not only the impact of geography on probation but also the consequences of widespread poverty and internal strife in a fragile democracy, all factors which ensured probation's low political priority. Connected with that has been a failure to develop an appropriate paradigm for practice and the pursuit of a patently unsuitable clinical approach.

A similar lack of homogeneity exists in the civil law countries. In Protestant countries such as Germany, the Netherlands, Denmark and Sweden the civil law tradition was tenuous while trading and political links with England were strong. In Germany, for example, British advice during post-war reconstruction influenced the development of both adult and juvenile probation. In such countries probation is the heir both of the Franco-Belgian *sursis* and of the liberal paternalism of the nonconformist Church reflected in the influence of voluntary prisoners' aid societies. In the Netherlands in particular the tradition, strong in France, of conflict between ruler and ruled which found expression in the 1791 Penal Code, and which so influenced the origins of probation, was no part of the cultural heritage. Accordingly to speak of the necessity of having safeguards against the intrusion of the state into the private domain would have little meaning. In Denmark the possibility of probation in lieu of the imposition of sentence has existed since the 1960s and prior to that, in a system perfectly comprehensible in common law, supervision was based on community involvement and control.

We see in respect of Hungary and the former Czechoslovakia and German Democratic Republic, that in Eastern Europe probation was welded on to a framework of communalism, and that this approach gave a new and literal meaning to the concept 'community correction'. In a barely professionalized criminal justice system operating in a context where the boundaries between the public and private were differently and more diffusely drawn, the idea of supervision by family, neighbours or workmates had a logic which enabled the former Communist countries to integrate their political and cultural aims with a western justice system.

That a change in the political system necessitated a radical revision of probation highlights the malleability of probation and its dependence on existing political structures. The Eastern European experience is an extreme form of changes to the nature and purpose of probation wrought by political change in Britain, the Old Commonwealth and the United States. What probation 'is' cannot be unyoked from the time and place in which it operates or from the political, cultural and historical 'baggage' it brings with it. As we argued in Chapter 1, few variables are constitutive of probation round the world. This malleability is one of probation's strengths, for it must reflect contemporary political aims and cultural norms if it is successfully to solve local problems of criminal justice and diversify the range of sentencing options available to the courts.

NOTES

1 In the United Kingdom the probation service has a complex structure. The England and Wales service is very large; Scotland (also included as a case study country) has a probation service integrated with its social work departments; and Northern Ireland, not included in this study, has a small but well-regarded probation service organizationally separate from that of England and Wales.

2 For a discussion of other more tenuous origins see United Nations 1951: 16–23.

3 Massachusetts Acts, 1878: Chapter 198: an Act relative to placing on probation persons accused or convicted of crimes and misdemeanours in the county of Suffolk.

4 A fascinating first-hand account of the politics of probation at this stage appears in Chute and Bell 1956: Chapter 6.

5 It should be noted, however, that the contrary view, expressed by Mr Justice Avery, that the phrase meant 'without proceeding to record any punishment or judgment' upon an offence which was proved was deemed by a government departmental committee of 1936 to be consistent with the intent of the legislation (United Nations 1951: 195).

6 It should be noted that this final criterion in particular is not quite clear. It is universal practice that the sentence is not executed in the event of successful completion of the *sursis*, but countries vary as to whether or not the original sentence is expunged from the record entirely.

7 Where supervision *was* involved funding varied widely, with the role of the Church and charities central in some countries, while in the Netherlands, Germany, Belgium, Luxembourg and Switzerland it was funded by an optional surcharge on postage stamps (Trought 1927: 125).

8 Ancel reports that in 1971 Denmark permitted partial suspension and Israel permitted only partial suspension where suspension had previously been granted. Italy, Spain and the former Czechoslovakia permitted ancillary penalties to be imposed alongside a *sursis*. In the

Spanish code examples given of such ancillary penalties are withdrawal of the right to hold public office or to vote.

9 *Département*-based courts of three magistrates, with sentencing powers of up to twenty years' imprisonment or fines of 200,000 francs.

10 Apparently all characters were played by London probation officers, one of them winning 'a special round of applause for his masterly impersonation of a defiant, loudly dressed "spiv"', and the script was also written by a London probation officer, John Burke (Page 1992: 227).

11 For accessible accounts of the rigours of the 'uniform' penal system prevalent in late nineteenth-century British prisons see (*inter alia*) Webb and Webb 1922; Priestley 1985; Forsythe 1987; for accounts of the failure of the approach see Day 1858; Balfour 1907; Priestley 1985.

12 This followed an abortive Probation of First Offenders Act 1887 (the political background to this Act is fully discussed in Bochel 1976: Chapter 1).

Part II

Comparative case study on probation services and practices

Chapter 3

Origins and purpose of probation

Koichi Hamai and Renaud Villé

This chapter presents the historical and legal background of probation services in the countries covered by the study, and discusses the aims, objectives and development of each probation system. The accounts of each country's (or state's) system have been compiled from the various reports prepared by the country experts. Countries are dealt with in alphabetical order. Two of the countries, Australia and Canada, have a federal structure; we have dealt with the former by presenting three examples of individual probation systems at state level and the latter by providing a generalized overview of provinces' arrangements for probation.

AUSTRALIA

The Commonwealth of Australia, created in 1901, comprises the six self-governing states of South Australia, Western Australia, Queensland, New South Wales, Victoria and Tasmania; the Australian Capital Territory and Northern Territories. Off-shore territories include Norfolk and Christmas Islands and, until 1975, Papua New Guinea (q.v.). Australia has taken steady steps towards self-government, receiving a large measure of autonomy from Great Britain in 1942 and virtually complete legal self-determination under the Australia Act 1986. Its population is ethnically mixed but predominantly white, though with a rapidly increasing East and South-East Asian population. Recent years have seen increased interest in Aboriginal peoples, both with respect to land rights and to wider aspects of discrimination (including their treatment by the criminal justice system), and significant legal clauses have been secured (Egglestone 1976; Hope 1988; Gale *et al.* 1991; Harris and Timms 1993b).

Probation in Australia should be set in the broader context of Chapter 2, where we outlined the export of the English common law tradition to countries of the Old Empire and its subsequent transformation under local cultural influences. Australian probation must be comprehended not only in terms of common law but as a development of the conditional liberty system introduced for early convicts, normally through tickets of leave. These origins, while they gave cultural logic to probation, sat awkwardly alongside the Christian reformism which drove probation in its salad days in England and the United States.

The subsequent transformations of probation must be seen in the broad context of Australia's increasing political distance from Britain. In contrast to the British situation probation developed slowly, and in spite of a well-developed juvenile system (United Nations 1951: 54) is in practice a post-war phenomenon. Yet while, as elsewhere, the concern in the 1950s was with meeting offenders' needs, cultural and political ambivalence about this aim caused the system to be slower to develop for adults than it had been for juveniles. In most states changes of name and administration occurred, the word 'probation' being replaced by 'correction', a concept which shifts the emphasis away from the passive act of 'supervising' (literally watching over) an offender on 'probation' (or being put to the test) to actively 'correcting' someone who has gone wrong. With that shift comes a further one, from a broad educational or therapeutic focus on the development of the whole person to a concentration on stopping specifically criminal behaviour.

It follows that in much of Australia probation is sanction oriented, but with the coda that the enforcement of sanction does not preclude change and growth. The shift from the Massachusetts position that probation is imposed instead of punishment to the idea that rehabilitation is a desirable but not necessary by-product of correctionalism finds echoes in other probation administrations round the world.

New South Wales

The historical roots of the New South Wales (NSW) Probation Service can be traced to penal practice in the UK. Forms of conditional liberty had been an integral part in the administration of justice from the beginning of the colony. Selected prisoners worked as assigned servants in the free community from the late eighteenth century. Good conduct led to prisoners' gaining 'ticket of leave' and eventually total freedom. The NSW Prisons Act of 1840, having both deterrent and reformatory aspects in which imprisonment was the major focus, laid the basis for incarceration for the next 110 years. Little sustained development in conditional liberty in NSW occurred in the nineteenth century beyond isolated, uncoordinated prison camps. NSW's prison system was reviewed in 1895. This resulted in the establishment of the Prisoners Aid Association, a voluntary agency which provided some assistance to prisoners released on licence and to first offenders when they appeared in court.

The basic framework of probation and parole work was created at the beginning of the twentieth century, though no specific legislative or policy developments in probation work occurred until forty years later. Following the recommendations of a commission appointed in 1945 and a Public Service Board report, the Adult Probation Service was formed in 1951 under the administration of the Attorney-General's Department. The Parole Service was simultaneously established under the administration of the Prisons Department. In 1972 both services were amalgamated into the Probation and Parole Service under the administration of the Department of Corrective Services (prisons). In 1991 the Service was renamed the Community Corrections Service, and in 1992 was moved to the administration of the Department of Courts Administration. The Parole Service was simultaneously formed, still within the administration of the Department of Corrective Services (prisons), and responsible for services to and assessment of inmates. In 1993 the Community Corrections Service was renamed the NSW Probation Service.

The NSW Probation Service's formally stated mission is to reduce the impact of crime on the community by effectively managing offenders and by being a decisive influence on sentencing. The Probation Service aims to contribute to offender rehabilitation, to community safety and restitution, and to the diversion of offenders from prison.

NSW is concerned to develop probation to restrict the growth of, or reduce, the prison population. The intensive community supervision scheme (electronic monitoring) is diversionary at pre-sentence stage. Community service was originally intended to divert, but has evolved through sentencing practice as another community-based option.

South Australia

The First Offenders Probation Act in South Australia was proclaimed in 1887 but was superseded by a 1913 Act which closely paralleled the English Probation of Offenders Act 1907. This provided for the appointment of voluntary probation officers, such as ministers of religion, justices of the peace and other citizens, and prescribed their duties.

In 1952, a Committee of Inquiry into the Treatment of Sexual Offenders recommended the creation of statutory probation officers. A juvenile form of probation was already well developed for offenders under 18 in the then Child Welfare and Public Relief Department. However, a political decision was made that there should be a distinct division between juvenile offenders and adult offenders. Consequently, the fledgling Adult Probation Service, which was formed in 1954, was attached to the then Sheriff's, Gaols and Prisons Department. Since then, the Service has gone through a number of name and organizational changes, and in 1991 was absorbed into the newly formed Offender Services Division which assumed operational responsibility for all offenders managed by the Department of Correctional Services whether in prison or in the community.

The Report on the Review of the Role of Probation and Parole Officers in South Australia, adopted by Departmental Executive in October 1993 defines supervised probation as:

> Imposed by the courts to give offenders an opportunity to demonstrate that they can be of good behaviour for a specific period. It offers offenders conditional freedom with the expectation that they refrain from offending and that they actively address their offending behaviour. It is granted on the condition that the offender accepts supervision by a probation officer and for this supervision to include elements of social development and social control.

The Department of Correctional Services' Objectives and Guiding Principles emphasize the protection of society whilst helping the offender. This protection is to be achieved in the short term through surveillance, monitoring and counselling of the offender; and in the longer term, through offender development, educational programmes and counselling to improve social competence and skills.

The 1993 Review of the Role of Probation and Parole Officers signalled the start of a trend away from individually focused therapeutic casework by the probation officer to a working method whereby the probation officer became the professional case manager working together with the offender in terms of assessing offender need, developing an individual case plan, implementing the plan by referring the offender to the appropriate service providers, reviewing the offender's progress, terminating the plan on completion or breach and evaluating the offender's response to supervision, as well as the quality of the services provided to offenders as a whole.

The early diversion of offenders from custody is becoming an increasing factor in Departmental planning of programmes and services for offenders under its management. For example, the introduction in 1987 of home detention (using electronic surveillance as well as social work intervention) as an administrative early release from the prison programme was prompted by concerns of overcrowding in the South Australian prison system. The Review of the Role of the Probation and Parole Officers 1993, now completed and in the process of being implemented, recommended that the Department target offenders at the presentence report stage, to encourage courts to use prison as a penalty of last resort and to promote the use of community-based sentencing options.

South Australia faces some unusual problems in working in very sparsely populated areas. In the metropolitan area the distance between the office and the furthest client is likely to be less than 30 km. In rural areas this distance is likely to be up to 200 km and in remote areas this distance is likely to be up to 500 km and requiring travel by air or four wheel drive vehicle. In rural areas the townships vary in size between 3,000 and 18,000, with distances between townships of between 30 and 120 km. In remote areas communities are around 300, with distances between 50 and 300 km apart. Travel in rural and remote areas is therefore a significant factor. With increasing urbanization, community resources in rural and remote areas have steadily declined over the years, thus adding to probation officers' workloads in filling the gaps.

Providing probation and parole supervision services for tribal and semi-tribal Aboriginals is difficult because of their high mobility between remote communities, because of the limited relevance of the concept of probation supervision to their culture, customs and laws, because of language barriers, particularly in the remote tribal areas and finally because of their special needs, which increase as they get further away from Adelaide and are more tribalized. Community service on the other hand has found a much more ready acceptance, with schemes operating in almost all tribal and urban areas. Aboriginals comprise 0.6 per cent of the metropolitan population and 2.3 per cent of the rural and remote areas. They are heavily over-represented in prison in South Australia, but are under-represented on probation supervision.

Western Australia

From the mid-1960s to the recent past the supervision of offenders in the community in Western Australia focused on the needs of the offender. Community corrections officers (CCOs) acknowledged responsibilities to the offender, the community, the court and the Parole Board or releasing authority ordering the supervision. In the event of conflict, the CCOs' first responsibility was to the authority making the order.

In 1989, the Community Based Corrections Division implemented a system of case management which features a classification and intervention model based on the offender's criminal activities rather than his/her assessed personal needs. The system, known as OSS (Offender Supervision System), involves the use of a screening device which focuses on the current offence and criminal history of offenders to determine a management regime which in turn determines the intensity of supervision. Offenders are subject to regular case reviews at stipulated intervals and within specified limits may have their supervision regime relaxed or tightened according to their compliance or non-compliance with the requirements.

The Offender Supervision System recognizes that a sanction-oriented approach does not preclude an offender's participation in services or programmes designed to effect change and growth. The divisional objectives make this explicitly clear. However, the community expects Community Based Corrections to be tough with offenders sentenced to its supervision. To the degree that Community Based Corrections implements this, it will be recognized and supported as a real and credible means of protecting the community and therefore a serious alternative to imprisonment.

In 1987, the Probation and Parole Service, then a part of the Crown Law Department, was amalgamated with the State Prison Department to form the Department of Corrective Services. Supervision of juvenile offenders remained with the State Department for Community Services. As a result of this amalgamation probation officers were required to consider issues of prevention and deterrence, in addition to the traditional issues of treatment and behaviour change. Prior to the amalgamation, probation officers had been required to have a degree in the social sciences, usually social work or psychology. This requirement was dropped with the creation of a unique employment category of community corrections officer, a recognized profession which was not tied to the pay and conditions of social workers or psychologists.

The amalgamation also led to the movement of prison welfare officers into community corrections. In recent years, sessional supervisors and contract workers (both are part-time waged staff) have been employed to supervise work and development orders and community service orders. Some pre-sentence reports are also written by contract workers.

In July 1993, the Department of Corrective Services was in turn absorbed into a larger Ministry of Justice, which has responsibility for services to both adult and juvenile offenders. The job was originally entitled probation and parole officer, but because of changes to the Service in the last five years, no staff deal exclusively with probation and parole orders. Supervision of probation orders now forms one part of the duties of CCOs, along with supervision of other types of community corrections orders such as community service orders, parole, work and development orders (fine default order), home detention and work release orders.

Prior to 1987 official statements set out the main purposes of probation as:

- to carry out court-ordered supervision;
- to assist offenders to resolve the problems (economic, personal, social, addictive, psychiatric/psychological) which

were associated with their offending, using casework and goal setting.

More recently, the officially stated purposes of probation have been:

- to monitor the behaviour of the offender;
- to put in place a management plan under which financial, addictive, psychiatric, psychological, health, interpersonal or other problems related to the offending behaviour are addressed;
- to supervise the payment of restitution in appropriate cases;
- to enable the offender to demonstrate that he/she will not re-offend.

The change from a needs-based 'welfare' or 'rehabilitation' model of supervision towards a 'justice' model has developed from a number of realities facing offender management world-wide. These include the relative scarcity of resources in the public sector and the concomitant demands for greater accountability in their usage, along with public demands for tougher and more decisive offender management. Recent years have also called into question the efficacy of the 'rehabilitation' model. It is difficult to define rehabilitation adequately, or to demonstrate whether improved social functioning of offenders, when it occurs, is the result of supervision, or is independent of it. Furthermore, many offenders have multi-dimensional personal needs, and any super-vision regime based on meeting those needs may be subject to more demands than can be met.

Western Australia is concerned to develop probation to restrict the growth of, and/or reduce, the prison population. A commu-nity corrections order will replace the existing orders of proba-tion and community service and will be of two types. One will be for minor offences and the other will provide for intensive super-vision and replace prison sentences of up to six months. The new order is expected to be administratively more streamlined, more flexible in allowing innovation, and more attractive to the courts. Recent new directions for community corrections include a greater focus on victims' needs and community involvement in overseeing the penalties imposed on offenders.

THE TREATMENT OF ABORIGINAL OFFENDERS IN AUSTRALIA

The descendants of the indigenous people who lived on the continental island of Australia before the first settlements of Europeans in 1788 have been described as the most imprisoned in the world. Whether this is true or not Aboriginal people are grossly over-represented at every point in the criminal justice process. The actual level of representation is not uniform at each point, however, nor is it the same in the six states and two mainland territories which comprise the Australian Federation.

Australia has a very broad definition of Aboriginality. Any person:

- who has some Aboriginal ancestry,
- who identifies him- or herself as Aboriginal, and
- is accepted by his or her peers or community as Aboriginal,

may be described as Aboriginal. Using this definition, approximately 1.5 per cent of the Australian population is classified as Aboriginal, but if one focuses on the adult population (persons aged 17 years and above), Aboriginal people comprise only 1.1 per cent of the total population. The difference is due to the relatively high birth rate and low life expectancy of Aboriginal people.

Even though the Aboriginal proportion of the population is very small, they constitute a significant element of the operation of all Australian criminal justice systems. For example, a detailed study of the numbers of Aboriginal offenders sentenced to prison and to non-custodial correctional orders found that 'for Australia as a whole, adult Aboriginal people are 15.1 times more likely than non-Aboriginal people to be imprisoned but they are only 8.3 times more likely to be serving non-custodial correctional orders'.

This study was undertaken by the Royal Commission into Aboriginal Deaths in Custody in 1990 and the report speculated that the reasons for the difference in over-representation may be 'due to a belief held by judges, magistrates and parole authorities that Aboriginal people are either less able or less willing to comply with the requirements of non-custodial correctional orders than are non-Aboriginal people'. The validity of this speculation has not been established, but a very comprehensive study of recidivism conducted over many years in Western Australia has shown that Aboriginal male prisoners are nearly twice as likely as their non-Aboriginal peers to return to prison within three years of first release.

An underlying factor which is widely accepted as relevant by criminal justice workers, including probation officers, is the difference between Aboriginal and non-Aboriginal lifestyles. Aboriginal people generally live very communal lives. Compared with non-Aboriginal people they are more likely to gather in public places in the open rather than in private, and if the gatherings involve the consumption of alcohol leading to boisterous and uninhibited behaviour they are highly likely to come to the attention of the police. Also, Aboriginal people tend to have large extended families, and are invariably hospitable to relatives and fellow tribal members. This can lead to overcrowded living conditions which may be seen as offensive to middle-class non-Aboriginal Australians.

Many Aboriginal people are highly mobile and frequently travel long distances to visit relatives. Those who live in a traditional manner have unbreakable obligations to participate in ceremonies, especially those relating to initiations and funerals, and these may involve considerable travel. Probation orders, community service orders and home detention orders given to Aboriginal offenders must take into account these aspects of traditional Aboriginal life.

With the exception of homicide, for which it has been shown that Aboriginal involvement as both victims and offenders is very high, as far as criminal behaviour is concerned there is no conclusive evidence to show that Aboriginal people commit more offences than non-Aboriginal people. However, it has been clearly established that they are much more likely to be arrested and detained in police custody. In fact, two national police custody surveys, conducted in 1988 and 1992, showed that Aboriginal people were twenty-six times more likely than non-Aboriginal people to be held in police cells. These surveys also showed that Aboriginal detainees were held in custody for longer periods of time.

The Royal Commission into Aboriginal Deaths in Custody lasted from 1987 to 1991 and investigated ninety-nine cases in which Aboriginal people had died in prison, police custody or juvenile detention between 1 January 1980 and 31 May 1989. No evidence of foul play by custodial authorities was found by the Royal Commission even though in some cases custodial procedures were criticized. The Royal Commission also found through its research that Aboriginal people once they were in custody were no more likely to die than non-Aboriginal people, the principal reason for the high numbers of Aboriginal deaths in custody being the high numbers in all forms of custody.

The Royal Commission made a large number of recommendations which aim specifically to reduce the probability of deaths
in custody and many others which aim to reduce Aboriginal disad-
vantage by improving Aboriginal health, education, housing
and employment. All Australian governments have made commitments to implement these recommendations and mechanisms
have been established to monitor the extent to which implementation has been achieved. The monitoring process has yielded
very little encouraging news to date, but a high level of public
interest together with regular and factual reporting of Aboriginal
involvement with criminal justice agencies is believed to provide
the best chance of overcoming the fundamental problems in this
area in the longer term.

(Written by David Biles, Former Deputy Director of the Australian
Institute of Criminology, Canberra)

CANADA

The Dominion of Canada, created in 1867, comprises the provinces
of Québec, Prince Edward Island, Newfoundland, Nova Scotia,
Ontario, Saskatchewan, Manitoba, Alberta, British Columbia
and the North-West Territories. Canada, like Australia, has taken
steps towards self-government, the last vestiges of British legal
control over the Dominion being removed by the Canada Act
1982. Canada's population is predominantly white, though there
are well over half a million native peoples, including 300,000
North American Indians, a much smaller number of Inuits
(Esquimaux), mainly in the north, and many black and other
minority immigrants from Europe and Asia in particular. As in
Australia, in recent years the treatment of native peoples has been
an issue of concern.

In probation terms as well as more generally, historical similarities exist with Australia. In both former colonies probation initially
followed the common law tradition (though in Canada much more
closely), was slow to develop, and really came more into its own
once probation came to be defined, non-therapeutically, as a framework for community corrections. Hence the 1960s and subsequent
years have seen a substantial increase in the use of probation and
the range of offenders eligible for it and a greater tendency to
recruit specialists as well as generalist officers.

Conditional release first appeared in the Canadian context in 1889. It applied to offenders with no prison convictions convicted of an offence punishable by at least two years' imprisonment. Rather than convict minor or young offenders, the court could where appropriate release them with or without surety, for a specified period of time. During this time the offender was to be of good behaviour and to make him or herself available to the court for sentencing, if required. Probation was mentioned specifically in the 1892 Criminal Code. In 1921 the Criminal Code was amended to include breach proceedings, sentencing options of restitution and reparation, and a power to order family maintenance payments.

A Royal Commission reporting in 1956 recommended further extension to the scope of probation work. In 1967, legislation extended the eligibility for probation to offenders convicted of any but the most serious of indictable offences, and provided an effective mechanism for dealing with breach of conditions. The current legislation came into effect in 1970, with only minor amendments since then.

Traditionally, probation services began as a service to the court. To this day the involvement of probation officers in the judicial process starts with the preparation of a pre-sentence report. The Fauteux Commission (1956) stated:

Probation is an alternative to imprisonment. It is a system designed to be used in conjunction with the power of the court to suspend sentence. It is, however, different from mere suspension of sentence. It involves compliance by the offender with specific conditions and his acceptance of correctional treatment under supervision ... probation is not leniency or mercy. It is a form of correctional treatment deliberately chosen by the court because there is reason to believe that this method will protect the interests of society while meeting, at the same time, the needs of the offender.

In Canada, criminal policy is established in the Criminal Code of Canada, a statute which is the responsibility of the Government of Canada, and which applies to all provinces. Provinces are responsible for the administration of the criminal policy as described in the Code. The administration of the different probation systems may vary, but the legal underpinnings are constant as a result of the national criminal code.

The general use of probation is described in the Criminal Code as follows:

> Where an accused is convicted of an offence, the court may, having regard to the age and character of the accused, the nature of the offence and the circumstances surrounding its commission, in the case of an offence other than one for which a minimum punishment is prescribed by law, suspend the passing of sentence and direct that the accused be released on the conditions prescribed in a probation order.
>
> (Section 737 (1))

Important legislative developments in probation can be expected. Bill C-90 was tabled in the House of Commons in July 1992. It died on the Order Paper prior to the 1994 general election. The new government introduced much of the substance of the Bill as Bill C-41 on 13 June 1994 and this Bill went to second reading on 22 September 1994. The Bill sets out a Statement of the Purpose and Principles of Sentencing. The basic thrust of the statement, from the probation perspective, is to place a greater emphasis on the use of sanctions in the community. In conjunction with the greater emphasis on the use of sanctions in the community, consultation with provinces and non-governmental groups is currently under way to improve the legislative framework in which the sanctions in the community operate.

In general, probation is not used explicitly to control prison populations. There has been, however, a general increase in the use of probation over the past several years, a period which coincides with increasing concern about the costs of corrections. This may also coincide with a growing understanding among criminal justice professionals of the potential negative impact of incarceration and an acceptance of the desirability of avoiding incarceration where other reasonable sanctions exist.

HUNGARY

Hungary's 11 million people are predominantly Roman Catholic and overwhelmingly Magyar; their language is one of very few in Europe which are members not of the Indo-European but of the Finno-Ugric group. Although within the Soviet Union interest sphere since 1946, from much of the time from the 1956 uprising until 1988 it was an intermittently reformist regime.

In Hungary probation is part of a penal code based on largely retributive principles, and is permitted only for crimes with a maximum sentence of up to three years. There is a dual system of juvenile and adult officers, though arrangements for probation are very loose: for example the Hungarian expert was restricted in her data collection because neither the president of the Association of Probation Officers nor any official in the Ministry of Justice (which has no separate probation department) could reliably answer all our questions.

Hungary does not at present have a unified probation service, and the juvenile and adult systems are dissimilar. The first Hungarian Penal Code – the Csemegi Code issued in 1878 – though very progressive by European standards of the day, did not have any provisions for probation. However, in 1908 the Penal Code was amended to provide for probation in the cases of juveniles as a care measure. Further development of probation in Hungary was retarded by the two World Wars. Statutory provision for adult probation was not made until 1975. The legislation enabled the court to order probation officers to supervise adults on release from prison. The probation officers were required to manage volunteers and to co-ordinate the work of statutory and voluntary bodies with an interest in offenders.

The work of probation officers was limited to the post-custodial supervision stage only until the next Penal Code in 1979. This gave probation the status of a measure in its own right, as well as retaining supervision for those conditionally released from prison.

The legislation specified the work of the probation service, set out the obligations and conditions on offenders imposed by probation, and regulated working relationships between police and probation services. This system is still in operation, with only minor developments.

Probation officers are employed by courts, each of which is headed by a judge, to use primarily interpersonal skills to report on and supervise minor to middle-range offenders. The academic competence of officers is high – all are graduates – but they are not trained or well paid. Probation officers have little discretionary power, and though juvenile officers have supportive functions, the work of the adult probation officer is mainly administrative. Nor is the idea of probation as an alternative to prison a political priority. In fact the court system in Hungary is in a difficult position: fines are frequently not enforced and the court system itself is so under-resourced that a gap of eighteen months between crime and sentence is not unusual.

The official purpose of the Hungarian probation system is to serve the public by controlling and guiding offenders, helping them adapt to society and by creating appropriate social conditions for this adaptation. The main responsibilities of probation officers are to provide the judge with information on offenders (at the judge's discretion if the offender is an adult but mandatorily if the offender is a juvenile), to help in sentencing decisions and to assist prisoners in leading law-abiding lives. Probation officers can also propose to judges that they vary the conditions of a probation order, extend its duration, or execute the suspended deprivation of liberty. Probation officers have to work in partnership with the courts, police, reformatory schools, medical doctors, local communities, employers and charitable institutions.

There is some mismatch between the official purpose of probation and actual practice, mainly as a result of current economic circumstances. For example, probation officers cannot readily improve the social circumstances of offenders. Unemployment is high in Hungary, and most of the offenders have no qualifications. They cannot work even in prisons, and on release from prison they have no money so they cannot even return to their home town. They are obliged to go to their probation officer, but the officer has no means of providing financial support for them, he/she can give only advice and inform the offender about his/her duties, obligations and responsibilities. Any contacts which probation officers are able to exploit in other organizations will have been built up through the personal attributes of the post-holder rather than by virtue of the post.

There is no formal probation policy in Hungary, the probation system (if indeed the word 'system' is appropriate) lies on the periphery of the judicial and welfare systems. However, some of the key bodies in the Hungarian criminal justice system are now helping the government develop proposals for improving arrangements for probation. These bodies are the National Association of Judges, the Association of Procurators and the National Association of Probation Officers.

One proposal is for a uniform probation system under the management of a national office. It has yet to be resolved whether this should be independent of the government (and from any kind of ministry) or a department within the Ministry of Justice. Most Hungarian criminal lawyers would like to see the juvenile and adult systems integrated under the control of the justice system, notwithstanding the practical difficulties in pulling together a system whose management is currently fragmented between five central government departments and local communities.

There have recently been significant changes in the Penal Code and related criminal policy. One such change has had a substantial impact on the work of probation officers, the abolition of 'reformatory and educational work'. This order was supervised jointly by probation officers and volunteers working for the same employer as the offender. That is one of the reasons why Hungary has no probation volunteers currently.

Hungary is concerned to develop probation in order ultimately to restrict the growth of, or reduce, the prison population. It wants to give a chance to first offenders and juveniles to reintegrate themselves into society without stigmatization.

ISRAEL

The State of Israel now has a population of just over 5 million. It was established in 1948 surrounded by the potentially hostile Middle Eastern powers of Egypt, Jordan, Lebanon and Syria. Ethnically Israel is very mixed, the Law of Return (1950) proclaiming that Jews from all over the world were entitled to come to Israel. Accordingly, in addition to almost a million Arab Israeli citizens and over a million Arabs in the occupied West Bank territories, the population comprises Jews from the Middle East and Eastern Europe (*Ashkenazím*) and Mediterranean Europe, North Africa (*Sephardim*, now comprising over half the population), North America and almost every country in the world where there exist Jewish communities. Official languages are Hebrew and Arabic; the *per capita* GNP is rather over a third that of the USA, Canada, Australia and Britain.

The probation tradition in Israel derives from its pre-war history as a British mandate and its original juvenile legislation from the English Children Act 1908. It has subsequently been heavily influenced by migrants from the USA. Its first probation officer, Reynolds, was English; its first social work department was instituted in 1944 under the British mandate and the same year saw the introduction of the Probation of Delinquents Order which, consistent with the common law tradition, ceased to regard probation as punishment. Though originally psychotherapeutic in emphasis, probation in Israel today does not continue this tradition: few of the probation officers are psychologists, most of them are social workers; all receive regular supervision from a senior social worker. The aim is to increase the individualization of sentencing and encourage courts to embrace rehabilitation-oriented modes of punishment.

The legal basis for placing juvenile offenders on probation instead of imposing punishment dates back to the mandate period and the Child Criminal Order of 1922, which was derived from the English Children Act of 1908. However, though the Order specified how to place a youth under the supervision of a probation officer, no organizational machinery was set up to implement the law. A juvenile probation service was established in the 1930s; and the Probation of Delinquents Order of 1944 reaffirmed the rehabilitative aims of probation, and specified in more detail the nature of probation orders. The relevant legislation was adopted by the justice system of the State of Israel when this was established in 1948. The Juvenile Probation Service was attached to the Ministry of Welfare, and probation officers, Jews and Arabs, who had been appointed since 1937, provided the basis for the new service and the separate Adult Probation Service that was established in 1951. The legislative provisions on probation survived broadly unchanged until 1971, when they were replaced by an Israeli law, the Youth (Trial, Punishment and Modes of Treatment) Law 1971.

Both the Juvenile and Adult Probation Services drew their authority from the Probation of Delinquents Order of 1944, which was amended in 1953, whose main points were:

- the court should not hand down a probation order without having first received the opinion of a probation officer;
- a probation order should be handed down for a period of no more than three years or no less than six months;
- probation should be considered not as a means of punishment but as a means of providing treatment and rehabilitation for offenders;

- the court could order probation only with the agreement of the offender.

In 1959, the Minister of Welfare published detailed regulations about the appointment of probation officers, the definition of their duties, obligations and rights, which are in force to this day.

In 1971, with the publication of the Youth Law (Trial, Punishment and Modes of Treatment), the courts began to impose probation orders. The unique feature of this Law is the creation of interdependence between the police and court on the one hand and the probation officer and youth on the other. Paragraph 12 of the Law states that if a criminal investigation reveals a basis for bringing a minor to trial, the police will notify the probation officer. In 1984, with the reduction of the age of criminal responsibility from 13 to 12, an amendment was added to the above paragraph, according to which a minor cannot be brought to trial before the age of 13, except following consultation with a probation officer.

The main purposes of the Probation Service are:

- to encourage the courts to develop a policy that places greater emphasis on individualization in sentencing. To this end, the Probation Service performs assessment work and submits to the courts recommendations related to behavioural change and rehabilitation;
- to modify the behaviour of clients in the direction of a termination of criminal activity; to supply the court with suitable therapeutically and rehabilitation-oriented modes of punishment;
- to participate in the legislative process with regard to the punishment, treatment and rehabilitation of criminal offenders.

One important development is community service, which is not necessarily combined with probation.

JAPAN

Japan, with a population half that of the United States and a *per capita* GNP some twenty times that of the Philippines, has a strong feudal tradition (officially abolished only in the late nineteenth century) and a reputation as a stable law-abiding society dominated by family values and corporate loyalty. Nevertheless these traditions have been shaken in the late twentieth century not only by a residual unease at Japan's role in World War Two (Japan regained full sovereignty only in 1952 and joined the United Nations in 1958) but by the social change and increased visibility of organized crime and corruption.

The operation of criminal justice aims to build on the community orientation of traditional Japanese modes of justice. Hence in relation to juveniles the Big Brothers and Sisters Association, which works alongside volunteer probation officers (VPOs), numbers some 7,000 teenagers (Rehabilitation Bureau, Ministry of Justice, Japan 1990: 21); while for the majority of adult offenders probation entails being supervised by a VPO, of whom some 48,000 are estimated to exist, in addition to over 55,000 juvenile guidance officers and many other citizen organizations which contribute to informal modes of social and in particular crime control (Braithwaite 1989; Moriyama 1989).

While aftercare services for discharged prisoners had existed in one form or another for centuries, it was not until the early 1950s that all elements of a community-based rehabilitation system – probation, parole and aftercare for both adult and juvenile offenders – was developed as an integrated part of a single public organization.

No specific community-based treatment system was implemented for juveniles until 1923, when the old Juvenile Law was enacted. The old Juvenile Law set up the Juvenile Tribunal and the Reform School. The Juvenile Tribunal was an administrative agency which handled juvenile delinquents who were not prosecuted at the criminal court. Having extensive discretion, the quasi-judicial agency was able to act upon the needs of individual cases with much flexibility. Including probation, it had at its disposal nine kinds of disposition ranging from simple admonition to commitment to the Reform School. Supervision in the field and in the hostel was carried out by probation officers, both regular and volunteer officers, attached to the Tribunal.

The present Juvenile Law was enacted in 1949. The Juvenile Tribunal was abolished. Its functions were broken up and taken over by three new organizations: the Family Court, the Juvenile Parole Board and the Juvenile Probation Office. Young adult offenders formerly handled by the Juvenile Tribunal were now dealt with by the newly established Adult Parole Board and the Adult Probation Office. The Juvenile Probation Office and Adult Probation Office were integrated into the present Probation Office in 1952.

Probation for adults in Japan involves the suspension of execution of sentence. Adult probation was initiated in combination with the traditional suspended sentence when the Penal Code was amended in 1953 and 1954. Supervision of those who received the suspended sentence was conducted by the probation officers attached to the Probation Office.

The Volunteer Probation Officer Law was enforced in 1950 to utilize volunteers officially in probation and parole supervision, formalizing the long-established practice of using volunteers in the rehabilitation of offenders. VPOs, though they are effectively part-time probation officers, are unpaid and have no conditions of service. Few VPOs are young (the average age is around 55) for they must be financially secure and have a good relationship with their local communities as well as sufficient time to devote to the job. They receive brief but regular training of a few days twice a year. Being a volunteer is widely perceived as bringing both satisfaction and status; loyal and effective VPO work can lead to public recognition through decoration. The work of VPOs, who submit a monthly report on their activities, is monitored by professionals; but while unsuitable volunteers can be dismissed, this is seldom done: it has not been found necessary and the disgrace would be great. Volunteers supervise the simpler cases, but if they become complex they are switched to professionals.

Japanese probation is the responsibility of central government. There are 50 probation offices and 900 officers, of whom 600 are in direct contact with offenders (about one for every 80 volunteers), all of them employed by the Ministry of Justice. Probation is administratively separate from parole; it does not have the job of reducing the prison population: prison numbers are culturally acceptable and there is no political pressure to adjust them.

The Offenders Rehabilitation Law (1949) describes the purpose of probation as:

> to protect society and promote individual and public welfare by aiding the reformation and rehabilitation of offenders.

It also describes the purpose of probationary supervision as:

> to promote the improvement and rehabilitation of the person under probation supervision, by leading and supervising him to make him observe the conditions [of supervision] ... and giving him guidance and aid, in recognition of the fact that he naturally has the responsibility to help himself.

The methods of guidance and supervision are:

> to watch the behaviour of the person under probation supervision by keeping proper contact with him, to give the person under probation supervision such instructions as are deemed necessary and pertinent to make him observe the conditions ... and to take other measures necessary to aid him to become a law-abiding member of the society.

The Law for Probation Supervision of Persons under Suspension of Execution of Sentence (1954) describes the purpose as:

> to observe throughout the period of their probation supervision and by prescribing the methods of such probation supervision and establishing the standards of its operation, pertinently to carry out probation supervision and help those persons who have been placed under probation supervision speedily rehabilitate.

It also describes the method of probation supervision as:

> guiding and aiding the subject person, recognizing that he naturally has the responsibility to help himself, and by leading and supervising him so that he observes the conditions.

Officially stated purposes are relatively consistent with the reality of probation practice. The effectiveness of probation supervision is beyond the minimum requirement level, as evidenced by the low recidivism rate of probationers during the probation period. However, the present situation can be improved on, and ways are being sought to develop treatment procedures and supervision techniques so as to reduce the recidivism rate even further.

Before World War Two, adult probation was conducted by voluntary organizations, whilst juvenile probation was conducted by probation officers attached to the Juvenile Tribunal, which was an administrative agency. After World War Two, both adult and juvenile probation was conducted by the probation officers attached to the Probation Office of the Ministry of Justice.

Probation officers for juvenile probation had been national government workers even before World War Two, while probation officers for adult probation became national government workers after it.

PAPUA NEW GUINEA

Papua New Guinea, annexed by Queensland in 1883, achieved independence from Australia in 1975. A tribal society comprising an ethnically mixed population of Papuans, Melanesians, Pygmies and other minorities, PNG has recently experienced a rapid series of political, economic and social changes, including a period of civil unrest in 1989–91 resulting from the activities of a separatist movement centred on the island of Bougainville. Social and political change has been associated with a growth in crime, and a probation service was introduced in the light of the recommendations of the Morgan Report (1979). With support from the United Nations Development Programme expert advisor, the Probation Act was drafted and passed by the National Parliament in 1979.

Although the Act was passed, no real attempts were made to implement it immediately due to lack of resources. In the meantime law and order problems continued to increase. The private sector through the Institute of National Affairs commissioned yet another study in 1984 to find solutions to the problem. This study team produced the Law and Order Clifford Report 1984, which emphasized the need for a probation service and community involvement in crime prevention and offender rehabilitation. The government then took action on this recommendation. Serious attempts commenced in 1985 to implement fully the Probation Act 1979. In 1986 the government accepted a 'Five Year Development Plan' for the Probation Service, which set the direction for the development and expansion of the system throughout the country. The Service presently has 22 offices across the country with a staff complement of 87 posts; there are also some 200 volunteers; and well over 4,000 offenders under probation supervision.

The Probation Act of 1979 provided only for an adult probation system. It established the positions of chief probation officer, senior probation officers and probation officers plus the engagement of VPOs, and it specified their duties. Generally the Act provided the legislative framework for the development of policies and programmes which govern offender supervision in the community and provide information to the courts.

After some years' experience of the legislation, the Act was amended in 1990. The amendment included lowering the age limit for probation from 18 to 16 years to include young offenders who were excluded from the Child Welfare Act and ensuring that the VPOs were specifically covered under the Workers Compensation Act. A third amendment was to enable courts to apply specific default penalties for breach of probation conditions, which again were not specifically spelt out in the original Act.

The introduction of the Parole and Juvenile Court Service meant a change in the organization's name from Probation Service to Probation, Parole and Juvenile Courts Service. Although the duties of probation, parole and juvenile courts officers are established under separate legislation, the same individuals discharge all three sets of duties.

The official rationale for probation is that it is one of the more economical, most efficient, flexible and adjustable methods of dealing with problems of crime. Although the Probation Act was passed in 1979 it was not until 1985 that the Attorney-General's Department began giving priority to the development of the Probation Service. The programme was implemented with the objective of reducing the rate of imprisonment with the following underlying basic premises:

- probation is an inexpensive alternative to jail;
- probation is a Melanesian response to crime especially in dispute settlement, i.e. compensation;
- probation is a 'grass roots' approach to law and order involving extensive community support;
- probation is correction in the community by the community for the community.

The Service's main responsibilities are to:

- provide information to the courts and Parole Board;
- implement and enforce community-based court and Parole Board Orders;

- design, provide and promote effective offender supervision programmes which involve the community in the fight against crime;
- safeguard the interest and welfare of juveniles in juvenile court proceedings and upon release to the Probation Service, their rehabilitation;
- work in partnership with non-government organizations on juvenile rehabilitation programmes especially in the juvenile remand and detention centres.

Legislation on criminal compensation, juvenile courts service and parole has yet to be fully implemented; once this has been done, no doubt probation policy will require consequent adjustment to reflect the directions the system will take. The PNG – Australian Development Co-operation Programme – Final Report of the Law and Order Sector Working Group (2 July 1993) proposed the increased use of community-based orders by the courts. Once the report is adopted by the two governments there will be structural changes to the PNG criminal justice system which could place probation centre stage between the offender, the criminal justice system and the community.

VILLAGE COURTS IN PAPUA NEW GUINEA

The introduction of state courts did almost nothing to maintain law and order among the indigenous people. In actual fact, the people encountered problems. Actions and behaviour previously tolerated by customary laws were outlawed by the newly introduced laws. Thus, the courts were viewed as alien and did not represent public perceptions and beliefs. In view of this, the colonial administration felt the urgent need to establish a legal machinery that would continuously refer to native customs and practices, thereby actively involving the people in the judicial processes. Village courts were finally established, but only after several false starts and considerable unproductive discussions and debates. The scanty proposals were prepared by expatriate officials of the administration for the indigenous society.

In British Papua, a system of indirect rule was implemented and the customs and traditional lifestyle of the people were clothed with legal recognition. This system, however, grossly failed to reflect the real structure of Papuan society. Ardent advo-

---

cates of indirect rule made continuous references to African experiences, where this system seemed evidently efficient. However, the fact remains that the advocates overlooked a significant difference. In most of Papua, a well-established systematic chieftaincy was virtually non-existent. Instead, a person was made a leader or chief because he possessed special skills, for instance, in fishing or hunting, that others lacked.

To overcome the obstacles, a law was implemented where indigenous people were appointed as customary judicial officers acting in the capacity of village councillors. They expressed the wishes of the people to the administration and interpreted the administrator's wish back to the people. The councillors and village constables bridged the language barriers and, more significantly, facilitated the administrative duties of the colonial government.

Indirect rule had yet another major setback, for even in areas of indirect rule, if a custom was found to be inconsistent with received law it was regarded as repugnant and not applicable. Thus, there was never a coherent development of customary law during the colonial administration. But notwithstanding this hindrance, the settlement of local disputes out of court flourished and proliferated.

Proposals were then made to establish native courts with jurisdictions to deal with minor civil and criminal matters relating to custom. Ordinances were then drafted to give effect to that purpose. However, despite the time-consuming genuine efforts that were made, the proposals were not implemented because of continued opposition from the Attorney-General's Department in Canberra and from some sectors within the then PNG judiciary.

The landmark development regarding village courts was made by L. Curtis and R. Greenwell in a special report that strongly recommended the establishment of village courts. A detailed report entailing recommendations on the establishment of village courts was then prepared by Deailly and Iramu, and the Village Courts Act of 1974 was a direct result of that document.

The village courts are the mechanisms for settling disputes and are referred to as a last resort. There are, however, also other methods which have been used in the community. The people go to village courts to seek external assistance when other informal methods of settling disputes outside a court fail to yield a satisfactory answer or solution. While village courts play a major role of arbitrating over cases, their mediating functions have been encouraged, and officials are instructed to mediate in every case before their formal powers are used.

Source: This information was extracted from the Department of Justice Village Courts Secretariat, Annual Report for 1988, prepared by P.B. Keris, Secretary for the Village Courts Secretariat.

THE PHILIPPINES

The Republic of the Philippines, comprising some 7,000 islands, was ceded to the USA by Spain in 1898 following the Spanish–American War, securing independence after the Japanese occupation of World War Two. It has a population twenty times greater than PNG but a lower *per capita* GNP. It is more ethnically homogeneous than PNG, mainly comprising Malays, though with extensive intermarriage with former colonial peoples, and therefore faces rather different problems.

In relation to probation the Philippines offers a combination of western individualism, constitutionalism, progressivism and correctionalism and an eastern traditionalism based on hierarchy and unified national purpose. In the Philippine criminal justice system the only sentences available are fines, prison and, once only and after a prison sentence has been passed, probation. It follows that Philippine probation is a pure instance of the suspension of the execution of, not imposition or promulgation of, sentence. No probation involvement occurs until the prisoner lodges a petition for probation, at which point the probation officer investigates to determine the petitioner's suitability.

Understanding probation in the Philippines, however, entails grasping a seeming dissonance between its restricted legislative basis and the character of its work. For all its seeming marginality to the criminal justice system the service has imported aspects of the American counselling tradition: probation is a graduate profession with supervisees termed 'clients', officers have a professional association and code of ethics, are paid more than teachers and police officers, and engage in individual, group and family counselling, as well as instructing their clients in civic duties, cleanliness and sanitation.

Probation was first introduced in the Philippines during the American colonial period (1898–1945). Act No. 4221 of the Philippine Legislature created in 1935 a probation office under the Department of Justice, which provided probation to first-time offenders 18 years of age or over, convicted of certain crimes. In 1937, after barely two years of existence, the Supreme Court of the Philippines declared the Probation Law unconstitutional because of some defects in the Law's procedural framework. A further attempt to establish a probation system was made in 1972; but the relevant Bill had not quite completed its passage through the legislative process when Martial Law was declared and the Congress was abolished.

In 1975, the National Police Commission, acting on a report submitted by the Philippine delegation to the Fifth United Nations Congress on the Prevention of Crime and the Treatment of Offenders, created an Interdisciplinary Committee tasked with formulating a National Strategy to Reduce Crime and drafting a Probation Law. After many hearings and extensive consultations, the draft decree was presented to a select group of 369 jurists, penologists, civic leaders and social and behavioural scientists and practitioners. The group overwhelmingly endorsed the establishment of an adult probation system in the country and on 24 July 1976, Presidential Decree No. 968, also known as the Adult Probation Law of 1976, was signed into law by the President of the Philippines.

Setting up the probation system in 1976–7 was a massive undertaking during which all judges and prosecutors nationwide were trained in probation methods and procedures. Administrative and procedural manuals were developed; probation officers recruited and trained and the central agency and probation field offices organized throughout the country. Fifteen selected probation officers were sent to the USA for orientation and training in probation administration. Upon their return, they were assigned to train the newly recruited probation officers. The probation system started in January 1978. As more probation officers were recruited and trained, more field offices were opened. There are at present 178 field offices spread over the country, supervised by 14 regional offices.

Probation is available on petition on one occasion only to prisoners sentenced to six years or less. Originally, those given prison sentences of more than six years were ineligible for probation. Legislation in 1980 extended eligibility to more serious offenders but – following a sharp increase in probation caseloads – the amendment was itself removed by Presidential Decree in 1985. This law also provided that an application for probation could no longer be made if the defendant appealed against conviction.

In November 1989, a new Administrative Code transferred the function of supervising paroled and pardoned offenders from trial courts to the Probation Administration. The Code also changed the name of the agency to Parole and Probation Administration in order to reflect this change. In 1991, the Parole and Probation Administration was assigned the new task of conducting pre-parole and executive clemency investigations in all city and provincial jails and preparing pre-parole reports for the Board of Pardons and Parole.

According to the Adult Probation Law (Presidential Decree No. 968), probation was established for the following purposes:

- to promote the correction and rehabilitation of offenders by providing them with individualized treatment;
- to provide an opportunity for the reformation of a penitent offender which might be less probable if he/she were to serve a prison sentence; and
- to prevent the commission of offences.

The preamble of the Adult Probation Law states that probation is intended as an alternative to imprisonment for offenders who are likely to respond to individualized community-based treatment programmes. The expectation is that all convicted offenders who apply for probation will be carefully screened, and only those who are qualified under the law, who are tractable and non-dangerous and capable of being treated outside prisons and jails, will be granted probation.

There are presently some bills filed in the Congress to extend the coverage of the Probation Law to include offenders sentenced to twelve years' imprisonment instead of the present ceiling of six years. There are also moves to amend or repeal Presidential Decree No. 1990 which provides that an application for probation shall no longer be entertained or granted if the convicted offender has appealed against conviction.

There is fairly close congruence between the officially stated purposes and the realities of probation in the country. As a less costly alternative to imprisonment, the probation system, after barely fifteen years of existence, has now under its supervision at any one time more offenders than the national prison system. Its revocation rate of less than 2 per cent is indicative of its effectiveness as a method of dealing with tractable first offenders. Probation is considered as a means of diverting selected offenders from residential or institutional facilities to community-based programmes.

Relieving prison overcrowding is a priority of the Department of Justice. Several agencies within the Department work as a team with the local government and jail authorities to provide legal assistance to remand prisoners undergoing trial, to expedite court processes and to help sentenced prisoners secure their early release through probation and parole. Probation and parole officers are actively involved in this programme by identifying sentenced prisoners who are eligible for the grant of probation or parole, conducting pre-parole interviews and submitting pre-parole reports to the Board of Pardons and Parole.

Another scheme for diverting offenders out of jails and prisons is the Village (Barangay) courts established in 1978 by Presidential Decree No. 1508. This law provides that petty crimes punishable by imprisonment not exceeding thirty days or by a small fine (of not more than P200.00), are no longer lodged formally for adjudication by the courts. Instead, the Lupon Tagapayapa or Barangay courts, composed of village residents elected by the people, settle their cases through conciliation or arbitration in lieu of lengthy and costly trials. The law has succeeded in relieving court congestion and has significantly reduced the number of petty offenders confined in the jails while awaiting trial. The Barangay court programme is separate and distinct from the probation programme, which has a different purpose and operates under a separate law. Nevertheless, these two programmes complement each other and have succeeded in achieving the common purpose of significantly reducing the number of prisoners confined in jails and prisons.

The Philippine Government does not provide public funds specifically for the rehabilitation of probationers and parolees, but it requires the Parole and Probation Administration to link up with other government agencies which offer these programmes and services. Such programmes as skills development, employment assistance, health care, education and social services are provided by these government agencies within the confines of their limited budgets. Non-governmental organizations supplement whatever government cannot provide.

In urban areas there are many private or non-governmental agencies and religious, educational and professional groups which give help to disadvantaged or alienated groups including offenders and ex-offenders. However, in smaller cities and towns, there are fewer community agencies/resources that can be used. Local government agencies, after having provided for the basic services of the community, have virtually no financial resources left for services to impoverished or socially disadvantaged groups, including offenders.

In remote villages, government services are very scarce. Probation workers have to be innovative and quite often must rely on existing indigenous social structures, institutions and mechanisms in the supervision of their clients. These include the traditional respect/reverence of village residents for elders or authority figures, the customary method of settlement of disputes and interpersonal problems through conciliation, mediation and consensus and the material and emotional support given to the offender through the extended family system which includes not only his/her immediate family, but a large group of close relatives and spiritual kin (godfathers, etc.).

SWEDEN

Sweden, a large but sparsely populated kingdom in Scandinavia, is twice the area of the United Kingdom with one-seventh the population. The population is fairly homogeneous, but contains over 1 million immigrants from Finland and more from the Balkan countries in particular. Traditionally liberal in social attitudes and welfare provisions, since 1990 Swedish politics and economics have become increasingly conservative, a trend from which penal policy has by no means been immune. The Probation Service in Sweden is located within a central government department. The correctional care system was reorganized in 1922, when the National Prison and Probation Administration was set up. This comprises seven correctional care regions, which are responsible for all remand prisons, local institutions and probation districts within their boundaries.

Swedish probation combines two traditions: the civil law system and a tradition of strong community involvement. Hence probation is a conditional sentence, albeit with 'a substantial degree of intervention' (Cartledge *et al*. 1981: 402) and with heavy reliance on members of the public (including ex-offenders) who, though termed volunteers, receive a modest fee (200 kronor per month) as well as expenses and compensation for loss of earnings. Sweden has some 4,500 volunteers – more than 10 for every probation officer. Uniquely, all probation orders are for the same period of time – three years – but normally involve only one year's supervision.

The Swedish Probation Service has its origins in voluntary associations, which were organized around the new county prisons in the latter part of the nineteenth century. In 1906, legislation established the conditional sentence. This provided for probation supervision as a substitute for a prison sentence, which would then be suspended. Supervision was carried out by police officers, or by volunteers from the professions, trade or commerce. In 1918, courts were authorized to call for social enquiry reports before passing a conditional sentence.

In 1942 the Probation Service was formally established. It started with 4 probation officers and 4,000 clients. Professionally skilled social workers provided a new basis for probation work, though they were supplemented by volunteer lay supervisors. In 1965 the Penal Code came into force. Sanctions specified under the Penal Code include imprisonment, fines, conditional sentences (penal warnings), probation and surrender for special care. At the same time, local Supervision Boards took over management of the Probation Service from the Prison Service. Reforms in the mid-1970s resulted in 66 probation districts staffed by a total of 439 probation officers, (plus chief probation officers and 250 clerical staff).

The main objectives of the Probation Service are:

• to contribute to preventing crime and preventing relapse into crime;
• to protect society;
• to contribute by means of supportive measures to clients' rehabilitation or social adjustment.

In 1983, greater emphasis was placed on the control function of probation. Supervision Boards were given a more formal and juridical decision-making role with regard to the restriction of liberty, special conditions, prolonged supervision, temporary arrest or revocation of parole. Chief probation officers were given more operational autonomy.

The government plans to extend the use of probation sentences. Probation sentences are to be given a clearly defined and well-structured content, so as to make them real alternatives to imprisonment. There are also plans to introduce new types of probation such as electronic monitoring.

The prison and remand populations are increasing. It is part of Swedish criminal policy that incarceration should be avoided as much as possible, since prison does not generally improve individuals' chances of readjusting to life in freedom. Furthermore, non-custodial disposals are more humane and less expensive than imprisonment. As a result, considerable efforts are being made to create sufficient confidence in non-custodial disposals amongst both the general public and sentencers so that they can be an acceptable alternative to imprisonment.

UNITED KINGDOM (ENGLAND AND WALES)

England and Wales are two of the countries which – alongside Scotland and Northern Ireland – comprise the United Kingdom. England and Wales share much the same legislative provisions, and have a single criminal justice system, which however does not extend to the rest of the UK. The population of England and Wales currently stands at 51 million.

The Probation Service has its origins in the work of the police court missionaries of the late nineteenth century, who provided informal supervision of offenders as and when asked by magistrates. The Probation of Offenders Act 1907 enabled petty sessional divisions (PSDs) to appoint salaried probation officers, and the Criminal Justice Act 1925 required them to do so, allowing at the same time for the combination of PSDs into probation areas. Numbers of probation officers have grown steadily since then, and probation areas have continued to amalgamate. The amalgamation process was at its most rapid in the 1960s and early 1970s; there are now fifty-five probation areas.

The roots of current probation work practice can be found in the spirit of voluntarism, often underpinned by a strong Christian conviction, which characterized much social work at the turn of the century. The guiding purpose of probation was, as originally conceived, to 'advise, assist and befriend' offenders who were in more need of help than punishment. Probation orders were not penalties in themselves, but alternatives to punishment; and the purpose of probation was to give offenders the chance to respond to a bit of straightforward commonsensical advice and guidance.

Probation practice became increasingly professionalized; the quasi-medical casework model of probation practice reached its zenith in the early post-war period, with the psychoanalytic movement exerting a strong influence. The 1970s and early 1980s saw a period of more marked uncertainty about probation work, as a professional and academic consensus developed that probation achieved little, or at least nothing more than any other form of disposal.

Since the mid-1980s, there has been renewed confidence about the scope for effective probation work. The Probation Service has begun to play a more important part in the criminal justice system. Central government has provided increased resources, and has looked to the Probation Service to provide a range of rehabilitative and reparative disposals. Whilst probation practice remains grounded in social work skills, there is a greater recognition that the Probation Service is primarily a criminal justice agency, and that the probation officer is an officer of the court. These changes have been accompanied by changes in organizational style, which has shifted from that of a loose network of autonomous professionals, to a much more structured and bureaucratic form of organization.

The Powers of Criminal Courts Act 1973 specifies, amongst other things, the duties and powers of probation committees; the financial responsibilities of committees, central government and local government; and the relationships of accountability between the Home Office, probation committees and local authorities. The Criminal Justice Act 1991 has modified these administrative arrangements, mainly with the effect of increasing the Home Office's financial and administrative control over the Service.

Legislative provision for the various court disposals provided by the Probation Service is scattered through several pieces of post-war legislation. The Powers of Criminal Courts Act 1973 consolidates the provisions for probation orders and community service orders, with minor subsequent amendments; more recently, the Criminal Justice Act 1991 has changed the basis of probation orders so that they are no longer alternatives to punishment, but a penalty in their own right. The 1991 Act has also provided for additional community penalties, for new conditions to be attached to probation orders and for the combination of community penalties in the combination order. It also extended the requirements on courts to consider pre-sentence reports before passing sentences, though subsequent legislation removed this provision.

Thus, as in Australia and Canada, there has been a marked shift in the perception of probation from a social work to a correctional agency, with probation officers subject to tighter local managerial control and managers subject to tighter national control. The incorporation of probation into court sentencing frameworks and the attempt to identify for it a firm position in the 'tariff' represents a shift from common to statute law, and the conclusion that the common law basis for probation has by the end of the twentieth century outlived its usefulness is unavoidable. In an international context of rising crime, the necessity of developing a non-prison-centric penal framework is clear, and probation's longstanding existence and the flexibility deriving from its common law tradition make it a prime candidate for administering such a policy; but the late twentieth-century preference for a mixed economy in both social and penal markets means that national probation services are less likely to be responsible for total service delivery than for functions of contracting, monitoring, managing and quality assurance.

The Probation Service Statement of Purpose, as stated by the Home Office, is:

- the Probation Service serves the courts and the public by:
    - supervising offenders in the community;
    - helping offenders to lead law-abiding lives;
    - safeguarding the welfare of children in family proceedings.
- the Service's main responsibilities are:
    - to provide the courts with assistance and information on offenders to assist in sentencing decisions;
    - to implement community services passed by the courts;
    - to design, provide and promote effective programmes for supervising offenders safely in the community;

- to assist prisoners, before and after release, to lead law-
  abiding lives;
- to help communities prevent crime and reduce its effects
  on victims;
- to provide information to the courts on the best interests
  of children in family disputes;
- to work in partnership with other bodies and services in
  using the most constructive methods of dealing with
  offenders and defendants.

The main purposes of probation, as formulated in these official
definitions, emphasize the rehabilitation of offenders and the
reduction of crime. There are several subsidiary purposes, shared
to greater or lesser degree by the Home Office, senior probation management and qualified probation officers and other
probation staff. In general, the Home Office has emphasized
the value of providing social work help as a means of reducing
crime, whilst within the probation workforce the view is quite
well established, especially below management level, that the
provision of social work help to offenders can be justified as an
end in itself. The diversion of offenders from custody is an aim
which until recently underpinned much of probation policy. This
objective was shared by central government and probation
managers, though support from main-grade probation officers has
not extended to the development of more punitive forms of
community penalty. More recently and particularly since the
enactment of the 1993 Criminal Justice Act, central government
has placed less emphasis on diversion from custody; but the
Probation Service continues to play an important part in the
criminal justice system.

Officially stated purposes are not fully consistent with reality,
mainly because central government and senior probation management are aiming to bring about a series of changes in probation
work which emphasize probation officers' role as officers of the
court and probation's function as a court penalty. There is
inevitably some conflict within the organization about the desirability of such changes, and inevitably a time lag in their
implementation.

OFFICIAL PERFORMANCE INDICATORS

Many governmental agencies have placed increasing emphasis on policy evaluation and performance measurement. Several have devised and introduced official performance indicators in respect of probation services. However, most of the performance indicators still largely measure work volume rather than the value of the output. There are no generally applicable performance indicators we found among the countries involved in this study. The following are the main indicators used by the countries:

- cost effectiveness (cost saving as a result of diversion of prison to probation);
- workload (caseload, number under supervision);
- success rate (number – rate – of successful completions of probation orders revocation rate);
- court satisfaction (court's percentage of accepting the pre-sentence recommendation).

Although among the above indicators the revocation or breach rate is most widely used, this is a negative indicator which shows the cases of failure. It seems to be important to invent some official performance indicators which can measure the effectiveness of the probation services both in quantity and in quality. The Key Performance Indicators (KPIs) used in England and Wales are shown below.

KPI 1: Predicted and actual reconviction rates for persons subject to community orders by type of order (which may be compared with reconviction rates for persons sentenced to custody, and to those fined or discharged).

KPI 2: Number of community orders completed satisfactorily (that is, without early termination for breach or a further offence) /total number of orders completed:

- probation orders,
- community service orders,
- supervision orders,
- combination orders.

KPI 3: Number of licences satisfactorily completed (that is without breach of licence including both breach leading to recall to prison and other breach)/number of licences:

- automatic conditional licences (ACR),
- discretionary conditional licences (DCR).

KPI 4: a Cost per pre-sentence report,
        b Cost per welfare report,
        c Annual unit cost/community order:

- probation order,
- community service order,
- supervision order,
- combination order.

        d   Unit cost/licence.

KPI 5: a Average number of days to produce a PSR in the magistrates' courts,
        b Number of PSRs provided to Crown Court within seven days of request by the court/number of PSRs completed.

KPI 6: Number of welfare reports completed within twelve weeks of date of commission/total number of welfare reports completed.

KPI 7: Number of occupied bedspaces in approved hostels/number of bedspaces in approved hostels.

KPI 8: Number of hostel residents successfully completing orders/number of departures.

KPI 9: Measure of court satisfaction (regular national sampling).

UNITED KINGDOM (SCOTLAND)

The origins of social work services in the criminal justice system in Scotland are similar to those of the Probation Services in England and Wales. Probation in Scotland also has its origins in the work of the police court missionaries of the late nineteenth century, who provided informal supervision of offenders as and when asked by magistrates. The Probation of Offenders Act 1907 enabled petty sessional divisions to appoint salaried probation officers. The principle is still enshrined in Scottish legislation that probation orders are not a penalty but an alternative to punishment.

It is only in recent years that professional social workers became significantly involved in providing services to the adult criminal courts in Scotland. For practical purposes this development began with the Criminal Justice (Scotland) Act 1949 which required the establishment of probation areas for every local authority burgh. This Act also initiated the system of social enquiry reports and gave clear authority and encouragement for the use of probation as a disposal for adult offenders. As a result of the Act, the Probation Service expanded rapidly and acquired increased statutory responsibilities including fines supervision and parole supervision.

The Social Work (Scotland) Act 1968 disbanded the Scottish Probation Service and abolished the title of probation officer. All the statutory functions of the Service for the courts and penal establishments were transferred to Scottish local authorities and local authority social workers inherited the role and responsibilities of the former probation officers. The main reason for these changes (outlined in the 1966 Government White Paper 'Social Work in the Community') was to avoid a multiplicity of services carrying out essentially similar work in the same community, or even in the same family; but it was also thought that the main function of the probation officer (personal social work with the offender and his or her family in the community) was basically similar to that of other social workers. The White Paper took the view that the body of knowledge and expertise required by social workers providing services in the criminal justice system was substantially the same as that of other social workers but added that specialized knowledge and experience were also required.

The Social Work (Scotland) Act also introduced a radical new system of juvenile justice called the Children's Hearings System. The central philosophy of this system is that children who offend and those who require care and protection are equally deserving to be considered as children in need, and that these needs should determine any compulsory measures of care. The system combines, within a framework of law, the best interests of children, professional (mainly social work) skills and the judgement of trained members of the Children's Hearings Panels who are drawn from all levels in the community. As a result, all social work services in Scotland were grouped together in single all-purpose local authority social work departments, and very few children under the age of 16 were prosecuted other than for serious offences.

The 1968 Act made no specific provision for the funding of social work services within the criminal justice system. Local authorities were responsible for funding all social work (with the exception of work in prisons); and during the 1980s, there was increasing concern that social work in the criminal justice system was losing out to other areas of social work, such as child care and services for the elderly, in the competition for funds. At the same time, it had become apparent that central government's criminal justice policies had not managed to control the rise in custodial sentencing. Scotland experienced a number of prison riots and an increase in the number of deaths of young people in prison. These pressures led the Scottish Office to introduce 100 per cent funding for the key social work services provided by local authorities in the criminal justice system, with effect from April 1991. Some criminal justice services, such as those relating to diversion and bail, continue to be funded from local authority sources, supported by government grant, but plans are now in place to incorporate most of these services in the new funding arrangements.

As is implied by the location of probation work within social work departments, the principle of community-based responses to crime in Scotland is that it should aim at assisting the reintegration of offenders, and as a result serve the interests of offender, victim and broader community.

The Prisoners and Criminal Proceedings (Scotland) Act 1993 introduces a number of provisions which have a significant impact on social work in the criminal justice system. It reduces the demand for supervision on release from prison by concentrating it on long-term prisoners (those serving sentences of four years or more). Most important, the Act introduces a new disposal called the supervised release order (SRO). This enables the courts when passing a sentence of imprisonment of not less than twelve months but less than four years to impose a period of supervision following release from custody where the court believes that such supervision is necessary to protect the public from serious harm arising from the release of the offender. The primary purpose of the SRO is therefore the reduction of the risk of reoffending, although the provision of support and assistance to those subject to an SRO by qualified social workers may assist the achievement of that objective.

Local authorities are now giving greater attention to targeting their efforts on high risk offenders, improving service quality in terms of its ability to reduce the seriousness and frequency of offending and the development of quality control systems. Inevitably, there are tensions between central and local government over such issues as levels of funding and the degree of central government influence over local government management decisions.

Scotland is concerned to develop probation to restrict the growth of, or indeed reduce, the prison population. Probation may be imposed by the court in any case in which it considers it expedient to do so – taking account of the circumstances and character of the offender and the nature of the offence. While not wishing to exclude the use of probation for minor offenders, the Scottish Office is seeking to concentrate its use, to the fullest extent possible, on offenders who are at immediate risk of custody and who constitute a serious risk of reoffending, especially those aged 16–20. Community service is restricted by law to those cases where the court would otherwise have imposed a custodial sentence.

Chapter 4

The probation order

Koichi Hamai and Renaud Villé

This chapter presents largely statistical information about the operation of probation supervision in the countries covered by the study. It considers what offenders are eligible for probation, the duration of probation orders and levels and trends in the use of probation orders. The final section discusses the sorts of standard and additional conditions which are attached to probation orders, and the arrangements whereby courts can revoke the orders when offenders fail to comply with conditions.

ELIGIBILITY FOR PROBATION

Different countries operate different criteria for eligibility, both in terms of offender age and offence seriousness. The lower age limit varies widely, as does the upper limit for offence seriousness. Although probation tends to be reserved for minor offences, it can be applied to serious offences in some countries.

Table 4.1 presents information on the minimum age below which offenders are ineligible for probation order. Where countries do not have a probation system for juveniles but permit juvenile offenders to be given probation under the adult probation system, we have regarded this as adult probation.

Table 4.2 shows whether countries use probation orders for minor, medium and serious crimes. Our questionnaire exemplified serious crimes as those such as rape, robbery, grievous bodily harm and the like; the examples for medium crimes were burglary and car theft.

Table 4.1 Applicability of probation order in terms of age

	Juvenile	*Adult*
New South Wales	—	18
South Australia	10	18
Western Australia	10	17
Canada	12	18
Hungary	14	18
Israel	12	18
Japan	14	16 (20)
Papua New Guinea	10	18
The Philippines	9	18
Sweden	—	16 (18)
England and Wales	10	16
Scotland	—	8 (16)

Notes: The figures in parentheses show the minimum age for probation in practice rather than in legislation.

Australia (South Australia)
The age of criminal responsibility is 10 years. The legislation requires that all offenders under the age of 18 are dealt with by the juvenile authorities for detention and community supervision. The Department of Family and Community Services is responsible for juvenile offenders. Offenders aged 18 and over are deemed to be adults and are referred by the courts to the Department for Correctional Services which manages the supervised bail, custodial, probation and community service programmes.

Australia (Western Australia)
There are separate services for juveniles and adults within the Ministry of Justice. A District or Supreme Court may impose an adult probation order on an offender younger than 17.

Canada
Probation services deal with both juveniles and adults although these are usually separated administratively.

Japan
Legally, the minimum age is 16 years of age. However, 20 years of age is usually the cut-off point in practice.

The Philippines
Generally, offenders below 18 years old are treated under the juvenile justice system whereby the court, instead of pronouncing judgement of conviction on the minor, merely determines the disposal and thereafter suspends all further proceedings and commits such minors to the custody of the Department of Social Welfare and Development (DSWD) or to bodies accountable to the DSWD.

Sweden
The minimum age of criminal responsibility is 15, but offenders between the age of 15 and 17 are generally handed over to the social welfare authorities for appropriate treatment. A person under 18 may not be sentenced to probation

unless this sanction is more appropriate than care under the Care of Young Persons (Special Provisions) Act.

United Kingdom (England and Wales)
A supervision order can be made on a juvenile aged 10 or over; the Probation Service generally deals with those aged 14 plus. Probation orders can be passed on offenders aged 16 or over. Young offenders (aged 17–21) and adults (aged 21 or over) are both eligible.

United Kingdom (Scotland)
A probation order may be made by any court in respect of any offence for which the penalty is not fixed by law and in respect of any person who has reached the age of criminal responsibility. The legal age of criminal responsibility is 8 years. Although children under the age of 16 are sometimes prosecuted before a criminal court, and can therefore be placed on probation, this rarely happens. Probation is available to the court for any adult offender unless the penalty for the offence for which he or she is convicted is fixed by law, e.g. at the more serious end – murder; at the less serious end – some traffic offences, etc. Probation and imprisonment are incompatible; that is, if an offender is imprisoned on one charge, he/she cannot be placed on probation for another.

Table 4.2 Applicability of probation order in terms of seriousness of offence

	Minor offences	Medium offences	Serious offences
New South Wales	Yes	Yes	No
South Australia	Yes	Yes	Yes
Western Australia	Yes	Yes	No
Canada	Yes	Yes	Yes
Hungary	Yes	Yes	Yes
Israel	Yes	Yes	Yes
Japan	Yes	Yes	Yes
Papua New Guinea	Yes	Yes	Yes
The Philippines	Yes	Yes	No
Sweden	No	Yes	No
England and Wales	Yes	Yes	No
Scotland	Yes	Yes	Yes

Notes:

Australia (New South Wales)
The probation order is used for serious offenders only in extenuating circumstances.

Canada
Probation is the most commonly used sanction for the following offences: sexual touching of a child under the age of 14 (89 per cent of all convictions); uttering threats of bodily harm (81 per cent); harassing/indecent phone calls (76 per cent); and sexual assault (75 per cent). It is frequently used for: assault; uttering threats of bodily harm: harassing/indecent phone calls; fraud under $1,000; and mischief (both over and under $1,000 property damage).

Hungary
Probation can be imposed when the maximum possible prison sentence allowed by the Penal Code is three years or less. Prison sentences can be suspended when the maximum prison sentence is a year or less (or, in special circumstances, two years or less).

The Philippines
A probation order can be substituted for a prison sentence for minor crimes and medium ones like burglary and car theft, provided that the prison sentence does not exceed six years. These will generally include such offences as slight or serious physical injuries, sexual offences, petty thefts, swindling. Offenders whose sentences exceed six years' imprisonment are disqualified from probation.

United Kingdom (England and Wales)
Minor offenders, frequently. Medium offenders (e.g. burglary, car theft), frequently, though special conditions are likely to be attached. Serious offenders (e.g. rape, robbery, grievous bodily harm), only under very unusual circumstances.

MAXIMUM AND MINIMUM LENGTH OF PROBATION ORDERS

Table 4.3 shows the minimum and maximum lengths of probation order (or equivalent) in each country. For most of the countries, the maximum length of probation orders is from three years to six years.

Table 4.3 Maximum and minimum length of probation order (in months)

	Minimum	Maximum
New South Wales	6	60
South Australia	—	36
Western Australia	6	60
Canada	—	36
Hungary	12	36
Israel	6	36
Japan	12	60
Papua New Guinea	6	72
The Philippines	—	72
Sweden	36	36
England and Wales	6	36
Scotland	6	36

Notes:

Australia (New South Wales)
Five years to six months are accepted by precedent as maximum and minimum lengths. However, there are technically no limits but all orders fall within the above range.

Hungary
When probation is a sentence in its own right the minimum length is one year, the maximum is three years (the judge has to define it in years), according to Penal Code No. 72. When a prison sentence is suspended and a probation order substituted for it, the order must run for the same time as the sentence for which it is a substitute, up to a maximum of five years.

Japan
The length of probation order corresponds to that of the suspended sentence for which it is a substitute.

The Philippines
The period of probation for an offender sentenced to a term of imprisonment of a year or less shall not exceed two years; where probation substitutes for longer prison sentences, the period of probation cannot exceed six years.

Sweden
Probation involves a three-year probationary period; the supervision is usually for one year. Release on parole, for persons sentenced to no more than two years' imprisonment, is usually one year.

LEVELS AND TRENDS IN THE USE OF PROBATION

Comparing the statistics of different countries' criminal justice systems is a hazardous enterprise, as definitions and methods of recording are bound to differ. Not every country taking part in the study could provide the statistics for which we asked.

As Table 4.4 shows, numbers of probation orders for adults have increased fairly consistently in Hungary, Papua New Guinea, Scotland and England and Wales. The trend for other countries is fairly stable, with the exception of Japan, which shows a fall. In most of the countries, the trend in imprisonment has been relatively stable, except in Japan which has again seen a steady decrease since 1984 (see Table 4.5). The proportionate use of probation orders and imprisonment is shown for 1990, in Figure 4.1. Traffic offences are excluded from Table 4.5 and Figure 4.1, except for South Australia.

Table 4.4 Numbers of offenders sentenced to probation orders, 1980–92

	1980	1981	1982	1983	1984	1985	1986	1987	1988	1989	1990	1991	1992
NSW	1,411	1,412	1,354	1,430	1,505	1,354	1,124	1,089	1,182	1,015	3,951	4,049	
South							1,836	1,936	2,086	1,979	1,146	1,277	1,295
Western											2,255	2,475	2,415
Canada							72,249	67,133	66,105	68,475	72,893	82,796	93,070
Hungary							3,565	4,037	7,574	8,861	7,126	8,987	11,908
Israel		1,033				1,310					1,505	1,566	
Japan	7,989	8,197	8,101	7,709	7,487	7,095	6,218	6,433	5,978	5,111	4,686	4,587	
PNG							668	918	1,262	1,676	1,304	1,882	2,076
The Philip.	5,577	6,629	7,883	7,469	7,627	7,728	6,985	5,476	5,234	6,317	6,670	6,517	6,927
Sweden	6,387	6,919	7,285	6,657	6,090	6,183	6,535	6,497	6,544	6,501	6,694	7,161	
Eng./Wales	33,600	35,850	36,810	37,950	40,080	41,750	39,690	41,540	42,440	43,280	46,282	45,593	41,369
Scotland		2,471	2,573	2,601	2,813	2,947	2,746	2,971	2,978	3,435	3,771	4,086	

Note: The following abbreviations are used in the table; NSW: New South Wales; South: South Australia; Western: Western Australia; PNG: Papua New Guinea; The Philip.: The Philippines; Eng./Wales: England and Wales.

Table 4.5 Numbers of offenders sentenced to imprisonment, 1980–92

	1980	1981	1982	1983	1984	1985	1986	1987	1988	1989	1990	1991	1992
NSW											6,160	6,565	
South						1,146	1,283	1,304	1,263	1,290	1,525	1,641	1,872
Western							4,344	4,583	4,408	3,977	4,988	5,385	4,179
Canada							119,299	116,269	117,325	116,051	115,100	114,834	75,156
Hungary							12,698	12,235	9,726	8,164	7,345	9,710	10,586
Israel		4,299				6,117				6,362	7,476		
Japan	30,232	31,888	32,957	32,063	33,648	32,988	32,207	31,071	29,317	25,910	23,608	21,993	
Eng./Wales	60,600	66,700	70,400	71,300	71,900	77,100	68,400	70,300	68,700	61,700	55,900	59,300	56,300
Scotland		10,419	3,333	13,602	13,693	15,519	15,292	14,110	14,243	13,645	13,000	12,041	

Note: The following abbreviations are used in the table; NSW: New South Wales; South: South Australia; Western: Western Australia; Eng./Wales: England and Wales. Traffic offences are excluded from this table, except for South Australia.

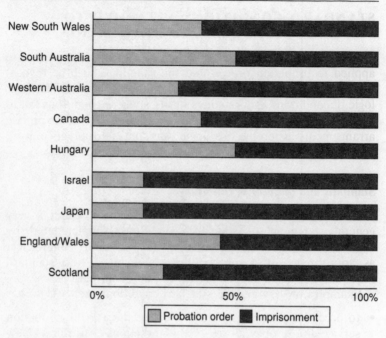

Figure 4.1 Proportionate use of probation orders and imprisonment,1990

Notes: Papua New Guinea, the Philippines and Sweden were unable to supply prison statistics.

Australia (South Australia)
Traffic offences were not able to be excluded from any of the data. Probation orders reached their peak in 1984, from when they declined by some 30 per cent in 1989. The current trend is a slow recovery.

Australia (Western Australia)
Figures for adult sentences are for financial years, from 1 July to 30 June. Figures for adults are orders, not individuals. Work and development orders are a secondary order, resulting from failure to pay a fine. They were introduced on 1 March 1989, with the aim of reducing the number of fine defaulters being imprisoned.

Canada
The significant drop in number of offenders sentenced to imprisonment between 1991 and 1992 is due to missing data from Ontario, that are not included in the count.

Hungary
The courts do not have to assign a probation officer to offenders who are placed on probation, and no statistics are available about the proportion who have an officer assigned.

England and Wales
Both probation and prison figures are for persons aged 17 or over sentenced by the courts.

STANDARD CONDITIONS ATTACHED TO PROBATION ORDERS AND REVOCATION

This section discusses the conditions or requirements that are applied to probation orders, and the sanctions, such as revocation, which are available in the event of non-compliance. The basic logic of conditions and sanctions in cases where conditions fail to be met was remarkably consistent across countries; but the precise arrangements whereby this logic was put into practice were diverse.

Standard and additional conditions

Most countries followed one of two approaches: either a very general statement of standard conditions, supplemented by a menu of additional requirements which the court could select as appropriate; or a much fuller statement of the standard requirements, again supplemented by additional options.

Examples of very general standard conditions are:

- to accept the supervision and the guidance of the probation service and to obey all reasonable directions (Australia – New South Wales)
- to obey the directives from the court or the probation officer; to maintain regular contact with the probation officer; and to keep orderly behaviour (Sweden)
- to be of good behaviour; to conform to the directions of the supervising officer and to inform the supervising officer at once of any change of residence or employment (Scotland)

Where countries had a fuller list of standard conditions, these typically included the requirement that the offender should report to a probation officer within a specified period (twenty-four hours for Western Australia and Papua New Guinea, seventy-two hours for the Philippines); notify the probation officer of any change of address; and report to the probation officer as required.

All countries except Japan had provisions for additional requirements of some sort. In several countries, the list of possible additional requirements included a 'catch-all' provision allowing the court to select whatever condition it saw fit. These included New South Wales and South Australia, Canada, Papua New Guinea, the Philippines and Scotland. Thus:

- the offender must satisfy any other condition which are related to his/her rehabilitation, and are not unduly restrictive of his/her liberty or incompatible with his/her freedom of conscience (the Philippines).

The main additional requirements include:

- medical and psychiatric treatment: e.g. Australia; Hungary; the Philippines; Sweden; England and Wales;
- drug and alcohol programmes: Australia; Canada; Hungary; Israel; the Philippines; England and Wales;
- financial compensation: Australia; Canada; Papua New Guinea;
- community service/reparation: South Australia; Western Australia; Canada; Israel; Papua New Guinea; Scotland.

Powers of Revocation

All the countries had some mechanism whereby probation officers could return offenders to court when they were in breach of requirements. In those (mainly civil law) countries where probation is a substitute for another sentence, such as imprisonment, the court's powers include the reinstatement of the suspended punishment (Hungary, Japan, the Philippines, Sweden). In (largely common law) countries where the probation order is an alternative to punishment, the court is able to sentence for the original offence (e.g. Australia and Scotland). In England and Wales, probation is no longer an alternative to punishment but a sentence in its own right; and thus offenders in breach of their requirements are no longer punished for the original offence but for the breach itself.

In many countries, the most frequent cause of breach is further offending. For example, in Japan 24 per cent of orders are revoked, and in England and Wales 15–16 per cent of orders are terminated because of further offending, but only 2–3 per cent of orders for failure to comply with other requirements.

Chapter 5

Organization and structure

Koichi Hamai and Renaud Villé

This chapter considers the size and structure of the probation systems covered by the studies, how they are located within the criminal justice system in terms of employment status, and probation officers' relationship with the courts. The first part of the chapter presents straightforward statistical information on each system; the second explores the formal and working relationships which exist between probation officers and the courts.

PROFILE OF THE PROBATION WORKFORCE

Table 5.1 gives an indication of the absolute size of each probation system, and its size relative to the population of the country

Table 5.1 Absolute and relative size of the probation systems

	Size of probation workforce	Population per probation employee
New South Wales	532	11,200
South Australia	184	7,900
Western Australia	224	7,600
Canada	2,750	9,900
Hungary	100	103,100
Israel	170	31,300
Japan	1,440	86,400
Papua New Guinea	88	43,700
The Philippines	1,272	51,600
Sweden	697	12,500
England and Wales	18,500	2,800
Scotland	950	5,400

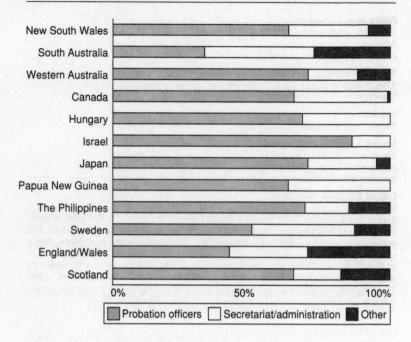

Figure 5.1 Proportion of staff in probation service

Notes:

Australia (New South Wales)
There are an additional 112 casual sessional supervisors in community service schemes. These 112 casual staff are excluded from Figure 5.1.

Australia (South Australia)
The Department of Correctional Services currently employs 184 full-time and part-time staff directly involved with community corrections work. In addition some 10 full-time equivalent positions are estimated to provide central administrative, research, personnel, supply and other functional support. The detailed breakdown is: 62 probation and parole officers; 8 district office managers; 11 senior probation and parole officers (primarily staff supervisors); 6 administrative officers; 42 clerical officers; 34 community service officers; 2 psychologists; 19 sessional community service supervisors (calculated as full-time equivalent).

Australia (Western Australia)
The detailed picture is: 166 (plus approximately 58 'sessional' workers); 95 of them (plus 58 'sessional' workers) would be described as probation officers, and 45 of them are secretarial/administrative. There is 1 clinical psychologist in the sex offender treatment team.

Canada
The detailed breakdown is: 53 headquarters staff; 171 supervisors; 57 senior probation officers; 1,634 probation officers; 53 assistant probation officers; 747 support staff; 20 other. No information is available on other types of staff, such as social workers, doctors and lawyers.

Papua New Guinea
The staff comprises only probation officers and secretarial/administrative staff. Although there are well over 278 VPOs they are not employees as such, and so cannot be considered as staff of the Probation Service.

The Philippines
'Other' staff in Figure 5.1 are: 6 social welfare officers; 5 psychologists; 2 doctors; 5 lawyers.

Sweden
'Other' staff in Figure 5.1 are: 12 physicians and psychologists; 12 medical staff.

United Kingdom (England and Wales)
There were 18,500 staff in 1992 (or 14,896 whole-time equivalents). 'Other' staff in Figure 5.1 are: 1,700 ancillary workers, 2,200 sessional supervisors and 900 hostels staff.

United Kingdom (Scotland)
Information about staff numbers is not collected centrally. The following figures are estimates, and the real figures could be up to 25 per cent higher: 450 qualified social work practitioners providing court services, probation and parole supervision, voluntary after care, community service and other direct services; 110 first line managers; 32 middle/senior managers. The 'other' staff in Figure 5.1 are: community service assistants (40); community service sessional staff (80); other community service staff (20); social work assistants (30). These figures exclude staff in voluntary agencies contracted to provided specific services for local authorities, e.g. hostels, day programmes, etc.

(or state) served by the system. It shows the total size of the probation workforce in each system, and the number of people per probation employee. Figure 5.1 shows the ratio between probation officers and other staff in the probation service in each country. In most of the countries probation officers make up at least half the total workforce. Staff shown as 'other' in the figure are generally ancillary or part-time workers, but we included specialists such as psychologists and doctors in this category.

Figures 5.2 and 5.3 show the proportion of female probation officers and the proportion of female management staff in each country. Scotland is excluded from Figure 5.2, and Canada, Hungary and England and Wales are excluded from Figure 5.3, as there are no data available. For Canada, we have used one of the provinces, Nova Scotia, as an example. In most of the countries the proportion of female probation officers is 50 per cent or more; the two clear exceptions are Japan and Papua New Guinea where only one in ten probation officers are women. By contrast, the proportion of women in management positions is generally less than 50 per cent, with the exception of Sweden, Scotland (the 50 per cent is an estimate) and Israel. Japan, Papua New Guinea and the three Australian states show especially low proportions of women in management positions.

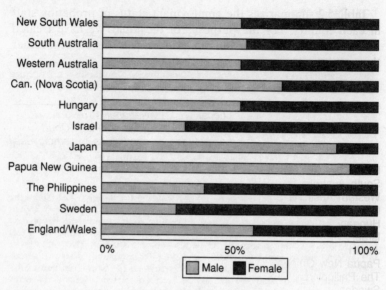

Figure 5.2 Proportion of female probation officers

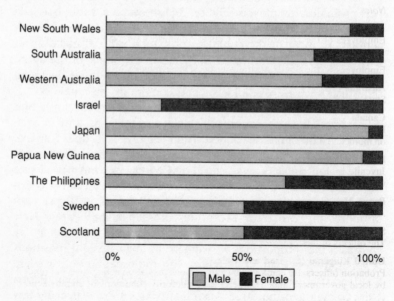

Figure 5.3 Proportion of female staff in management positions

Table 5.2 summarizes the employment status of probation staff in each country. For the purposes of the table, we have treated Australian states and Canadian provinces as forms of local rather than central government.

Table 5.2 Employment status of probation staff

	Local government employees	National government employees	Court employees
New South Wales	X		
South Australia	X		
Western Australia	X		
Canada	X		
Hungary			X
Israel		X	
Japan		X	
Papua New Guinea		X	
The Philippines		X	
Sweden	X		
England and Wales	X		
Scotland	X		

Notes:

Australia (New South Wales)
Employees of the Department of Courts Administration, NSW government.

Australia (South Australia)
Employees of the South Australia Justice Department.

Australia (Western Australia)
State government employees.

Canada
Probation officers are employed by provincial governments (rather than federal or municipal government).

Hungary
Juvenile probation officers are employed by local authorities, and those dealing with adults, by county courts.

Papua New Guinea
All probation staff are national government employees.

Sweden
The officers of the Swedish probation service are central government civil servants.

United Kingdom (England and Wales)
Probation officers are employed by autonomous probation committees but funded by local government under (largely) local authority conditions of employment.

United Kingdom (Scotland)
Probation work is done by social workers employed by local government.

PROBATION OFFICERS AND THE COURT

The rest of this chapter examines, on a country-by-country basis, the balance struck in different systems between being 'servants of the court' and 'professional advisers', the role probation officers play in providing sentencers with court reports giving advice and information, and the value placed by sentencers on such advice.

Relationships between courts and probation officers are in general complicated ones, in that probation officers in most of the countries in the study provide services to sentencers and are accountable to the court, but are neither employees of the court nor formally contracted to the court. The provision of advice to the courts is a function performed by most of the systems covered by the study; however, this role is often not of disinterested advisor, but of advocate of probation disposals: probation reports in some systems by convention propose only probation or other community penalties to the court.

Australia (New South Wales)

Probation officers are not directly employed by the courts but could be described as 'officers of the court' in carrying out any request or direction of the court. There is a statutory requirement upon sentencers to obtain an assessment of suitability for community service and periodic detention. The purpose of a pre-sentence report is to provide the court with information about the offender which may be taken into account in determining an appropriate sentence. Reports contain background information regarding the offender's history and circumstances, including family, social and employment-related information. The offender's attitude to the offence and the context of the offending behaviour is presented. The report ends with an assessment of the offender's suitability for programmes supervised by the Service. In cases where the offender presents a significant risk to the community and should be imprisoned, then such an assessment is appropriate for inclusion in the report.

Sentencers generally find pre-sentence reports useful in determining an appropriate sentence, particularly when non-custodial sanctions are contemplated.

Australia (South Australia)

Probation officers are not employed by the courts, however they prepare reports for the courts and supervise offenders on court-imposed orders. Their role is that of 'professional advisers'. The pre-sentence reports prepared by probation officers are intended to help the court decide on an appropriate sentence. An evaluation of the appropriateness of the various community-based sentencing options is included in every report. Custodial sentences are not proposed in reports although comments on the negative effects of imprisonment may be included in some instances. Reports tend not to advise courts on sentences other than probation-related ones, although this is only by custom.

Australia (Western Australia)

Community corrections officers are employed by the state government, but a statutory reporting requirement gives them dual status as officers of the court. They are required to provide objective advice to the court regarding dispositions being considered, and carry out the orders of the court.

Community corrections officers advise the court on a range of sentencing options from good behaviour bonds through to the likelihood of an offender responding to parole. Reports are requested for around half of offenders being sentenced in the higher courts (District and Supreme). Judges are thought to follow the recommendations made by community corrections officers in about two-thirds of cases.

Canada

Though the federal government has exclusive jurisdiction over legislation on criminal matters, provincial governments have exclusive authority over the administration of the criminal law within their respective jurisdictions. The provision of court services to both adult and young offenders falls generally within the jurisdiction of the provinces, though prison sentences of two years and over are the responsibility of the federal government.

Probation officers are employees of the provincial government with responsibility for administering the law in that province. The court does not employ probation officers but probation officers are usually considered to be officers of the court. (In Nova Scotia, however, the Chief Provincial Court Judge has taken the position that probation officers are not officers of the court unless they have been designated as such by the court.)

Probation officers can be asked by the court to provide written pre-sentence reports where offenders have pleaded guilty, or been found guilty, of an offence. The reports are to help the court in passing sentence or in determining whether the accused should be discharged. Whether pre-sentence reports include a recommendation on sentence varies from jurisdiction to jurisdiction, and even from judge to judge. PSRs may recommend conditions, either general or special, which the court may want to consider. If probation is granted, the probation officer will carry out the order of the court.

Hungary

The county courts employ probation officers. Where probation orders are made, the judge gives his or her instructions to the probation officer when passing sentence. There are standard requirements for probation supervision specified by the Penal Code and related decrees, to which the judge can add other special requirements. Probation officers are not 'servants of the court', they are 'servants of society', because their purpose is to protect society from crimes mainly by prevention. They have no role in providing sentencers with advice.

Israel

Probation officers have organizational and professional autonomy and they are part of the Labour and Welfare Affairs Ministry. They serve the courts and law enforcement agencies in the capacity of professional advisors, and are so recognized by the courts and treatment-rehabilitation agencies.

Japan

The Probation Office is an administrative organization, located within the Ministry of Justice, and is completely independent from the courts, which form a judicial organization. Courts decide whether or not to make a probation order, and when they do the execution of the court's decision is the responsibility of the Probation Office of the Ministry of Justice.

Papua New Guinea

Although probation officers are 'officers of the court' they are not employed by the courts. Courts have no authority to direct the work of probation officers. Probation officers from chief probation officer (CPO) downwards are appointed by central government. All staff are accountable to the CPO and in turn the CPO is accountable to the Deputy Secretary of the Department of the Attorney General.

Courts may request pre-sentence reports from the Probation Service, and probation officers prepare these. When preparing PSRs the main task of the probation officers is to assist the courts towards determining the most suitable method of dealing with an offender. These PSRs are expected to contain the offender's personal history, his/her views on the offence committed plus views from his/her family and relatives, the victim and relatives and community generally. Reports should also indicate how the matter could be settled locally. The only recommendation contained in the report is on whether the offender is suitable or not for probation supervision. Courts do not accept probation officers making recommendations for other sentences.

The Philippines

Probation and parole officers are appointed by the Parole and Probation Administration. Each probation field office is headed by a chief parole and probation officer (CPPO) to whom the subordinate officers report. The CPPO, in turn, is directly responsible to a regional director.

Applications for probation are filed by the offender with the trial court which convicted him or her. If the application is accepted, the court issues an order to the probation office to conduct a post-sentence investigation and to submit a report within sixty days from the date the order is received. The court has to act on the report within fifteen days upon receipt thereof. If probation is granted, the court issues another order to the probation office to supervise the probationer for a period set by the court. During the supervision period, the probation and parole officer may, on behalf of the probationer, request the court for modification of conditions of probation, change of residence, permission to travel.

The conditions of probation as well as the length of the supervision period imposed by the court define the limits within which probation treatment takes place. These conditions may be regarded as the instruction of the court to both the probation officer and the probationer as to how probation supervision should be conducted.

Sweden

The duties and responsibilities of prosecutors and courts are laid down in law as are those of the probation authorities. Each of these is responsible and accountable under the law. The probation service is, however, an independent agency for which no judicial authority as such has administrative or managerial responsibility. A variety of judicial and administrative procedures exists to check whether the probation authorities have discharged their responsibilities correctly and, should this not be the case, to determine the action to be taken. Naturally, however, effective probation work presupposes contact with prosecutors and courts in order to ensure adequate exchange of information and the building of relations of mutual respect and understanding. The introduction of community service has led to the setting-up of joint consultation groups (which also include defence lawyers, police, etc.) for regular exchange of information.

United Kingdom (England and Wales)

Probation officers are 'officers of the court' and prepare reports for magistrates and supervise offenders under various orders. However, they are not employed directly by the court, and individual magistrates have no authority to direct the work of probation officers. The Probation Committee (two-thirds of whose members are magistrates) appoints a chief probation officer, to whom probation officers are accountable.

The main task of probation officers when preparing pre-sentence reports for sentencers (whether magistrates or judges) is to help the court in determining the most suitable method of dealing with an offender. Reports are expected to contain, wherever relevant, a proposal for the most suitable community sentence. By convention, reports never propose a custodial sentence (even if they sometimes imply the inevitability of this); but they sometimes suggest sentences other than probation-related ones.

Sentencers generally say that they find pre-sentence reports valuable in reaching in a sentencing decision. This is especially true for lay magistrates; in a recent survey only 5 per cent said that they did not find them useful.

United Kingdom (Scotland)

Local authority social work departments are accountable to their own regional or island council for the provision of services to the criminal courts and, ultimately, to the Secretary of State. They are legally required to provide information and advice to courts as an aid to sentencing as well as those services which the court requires for dealing with offenders in the community wherever possible. Staff providing these services are not therefore 'servants of the court' and do not receive 'instructions' from the court. They are accountable to the court for the accuracy of the information they provide, and for the soundness of any conclusions/ advice/recommendations they make as an aid to sentencing. They are also accountable for the general standard of the services they provide on behalf of the court in respect of court disposals involving social work intervention: in this respect they act as 'agents' rather than 'officers' of the court. Sentencers need to be assured of precisely what service will be provided when they make an order involving social work services or request information and advice to assist sentencing. They also need assurance that high quality services will be provided, and that standards will be rigorously applied and effectively administered by suitably qualified staff, if their confidence in these services is to be maintained. National Standards provide a framework of policy and practice guidance for this purpose. These National Standards also set out arrangements for liaison between local services and sentencers in local courts which are designed to deal both with day-to-day problems and with more strategic issues relating to the nature and quality of the service provided. Liaison arrangements of this kind are now standard practice in all authorities.

Only qualified social workers provide information and advice to the courts on sentencing. That advice is aimed at helping the court to determine the most suitable method of dealing with the offender. Such advice may cover the full range of community-based disposals. Report writers are expected to concentrate on making feasible community-based options available to the court especially where there is an immediate risk of a custodial sentence or of further offending. If the report writer has a preferred option this should be recommended. Where a report writer has no recommendation to make, this must be stated and the reasons given. Most sentencers welcome recommendations, some do not. Courts sometimes ask for particular problems or particular social work disposals to be considered when requesting a social enquiry report, although this is not a general practice and some sentencers resist it.

Reports are requested on offenders who, because of the seriousness of the current offence and/or previous offending, face an almost inevitable custodial sentence. Report writers may acknowledge this likelihood but are not expected by National Standards to recommend custody. Even in such cases they should offer a feasible alternative, if there is one. Since October 1993 those writing reports for courts where a custodial sentence seems inevitable have, in addition, been required to consider whether a supervised release order might be appropriate.

Sentencers generally say that they find social enquiry reports a valuable service in reaching sentencing decisions.

Chapter 6

Probation as a profession

Koichi Hamai and Renaud Villé

The claims made by various occupational groups to be members of the professions are usually grounded on at least one of the following features: self-regulation through codes of practice; entry qualifications (or training) at tertiary academic level; a well-documented body of knowledge and skills; and clearly established career progression. In probation as in other occupations there are clear pressures for greater professional status, but at the same time there are countervailing 'managerialist' pressures in some of the countries examined intended to render probation work more consistent with the broader objectives of the criminal justice system within which they are located. This chapter considers the extent to which each probation system is 'professionalised' and assesses where probation officers in each system are located in the employment market.

PROFESSIONAL ASSOCIATIONS AND TRADE UNIONS

Table 6.1 shows whether each system has a professional association, a code of ethics and a union. The table, read together with the explanatory notes, makes it clear that a professional association is available to probation officers in most of the twelve probation systems. In seven systems this association is either one specifically for probation officers or else for social workers and probation officers. In several countries the professional association also serves as a trade union, negotiating with employing bodies over pay and conditions of service. Only four systems have formal codes of ethics specifically for probation work.

Table 6.1 Association, union and code of ethics

	Association	Union	Code of ethics
New South Wales	X	X	Yes
South Australia	X	X	No
Western Australia			No
Canada			Yes
Hungary	X		No
Israel	X	X	Yes
Japan		X	No
Papua New Guinea			No
The Philippines	X		Yes
Sweden	X	X	No
England and Wales	X		No
Scotland	X	X	Yes

Notes:

Australia (New South Wales)
Membership of the professional association stands at 65 per cent and of the staff union at 70 per cent.

Australia (South Australia)
About 40 per cent of eligible probation and parole officers are members of the South Australian Probation and Parole Officers' Association. The Probation and Parole Officers' Association does not have a code of ethics. However, all probation and parole officers are expected to work in accordance with the Departmental Mission Statement, its Strategic Directions and its Statement of Beliefs. In addition a number of probation and parole officers are members of the Australian Association of Social Workers, the national professional accreditation body for social workers. (Probation officers are required to be qualified social workers and are therefore bound by the ethics of that profession.)

Australia (Western Australia)
Officers can join the State Civil Service Association. CCOs are governed by the same rules as other public servants. Professional ethics also guide officers if they have professional affiliations such as social work or psychology. CCOs are bound by the confidentiality rules set out in Section 51 of the Offenders Probation and Parole Act.

Canada
There are some associations of probation officers, notably in Ontario, Nova Scotia and New Brunswick. One-third to one-half of officers are members of these associations. Ontario has a code of ethics, established by the Probation Officers Association of Ontario. There is no national association.

Hungary
The National Association of Hungarian Probation Officers is a professional association which also acts as a union. It represents all the adult probation officers.

Israel
There is a Voluntary Association within the Social Work Union. All probation officers are members of this Association. The Social Work Union has its own code of ethics.

Japan
There is no association and/or union specifically for probation officers. Probation officers can join the Staff Union for National Civil Servants. There is a code of ethics for all government officials.

Papua New Guinea
Although there are no code of ethics or guidelines for probation officers to follow, the Probation Service's policy and operations manual contains the rules and standards expected from all staff within the organization.

The Philippines
The Parole and Probation Officers' League of the Philippines (PPOLP), Inc. is open to probation officers and other staff. There is a Code of Conduct and Ethical Standards mandated by law for all public officials and employees in the Philippine Government (Republic Act No. 6713).

Sweden
Fifty per cent of probation officers and almost all ancillary workers are members of the Swedish Central Organization of Salaried Employees. This represents probation officers, assistant chief officers and chief officers in negotiations on pay and conditions of service with employers and also represents these groups on professional matters. About half of probation officers, assistant chief officers and chief officers belong to the union, the Swedish Confederation of Professional Associations (SACO). The role of SACO is to represent the economic, academic and professional interests of individual members.

United Kingdom (England and Wales)
The National Association of Probation Officers performs the function both of a professional association and of a trade union for probation officers and ancillary workers. About two-thirds of eligible staff are members; it has a national headquarters and local branches corresponding to probation areas. The Association of Chief Officers of Probation is the professional association for senior managers. There is also the Probation Managers' Association, a professional association for senior probation officers, with about a third of the eligible membership.

United Kingdom (Scotland)
The British Association of Social Workers (BASW) is the largest professional association representing social work practitioners in Scotland. UNISON is the trade union for all local authority staff including those working in the criminal justice system. The Association of Directors of Social Work (ADSW) is the professional association of senior social work management in local authorities – down to third tier level. It has a Standing Committee on Social Work Services in the Criminal Justice System on which many of those with responsibility for offender services at middle management level are co-opted members. BASW has some 1,000 members in Scotland (about one-third of all practitioners); most practitioners are members of UNISON; only a handful of those who manage offender services are senior enough to qualify for membership of ADSW.

CODE OF ETHICS (PRINCIPLES OF PRACTICE) OF THE PROBATION AND PAROLE OFFICERS' ASSOCIATION (NEW SOUTH WALES, AUSTRALIA)

All members of this Association understand that they will:

a   Respect the inherent dignity and worth of every human being and seek to ensure that, within the scope of their work, the offender's human and civil liberties are safeguarded.

b   Treat all offenders without prejudice.

c   Help offenders to increase their range of legitimate options and encourage them to take responsibility for their own actions.

d   Be supportive and non-judgemental even when obliged to protect others from the offender, or when dealing with non-co-operative offenders or when acknowledging an inability to help an offender.

e   Recognize the need to work with others for effectiveness, and the limits of one's competence and authority.

f   Accept that education, training, support and supervision are basic to the work of the probation and parole officer and hold themselves responsible for the standard of their work with offenders.

g   Acknowledge the responsibility to help offenders obtain the services and rights to which they are entitled.

h   Respect the privacy of those supervised and contacted in the course of work and of the information about them.

i   Show respect for the courts, the department and government and not knowingly give incorrect information, or advice, which is to their knowledge contrary to the law.

j   Make clear in any public statement whether they are acting in a personal capacity or on behalf of an organization.

k   Treat colleagues and others supportively and with courtesy and fairness.

l   Contribute to the formation and implementation of policies of justice, corrections and welfare which will improve both the lifestyle and the functioning of the community.

m   Work for the creation and maintenance in the criminal justice field of conditions which will enable officers to accept the responsibilities of this code of ethics.

Source: Probation and Parole Officers' Association (New South Wales, Australia)

THE PROFESSIONAL ASSOCIATION FOR PROBATION OFFICERS IN THE PHILIPPINES

The functions of the Association, spelt out in Article II of its Constitution and By-laws entitled Objectives and Purposes, are:

* To promote a respectable, honest competent, efficient and effective parole and probation service;
* To establish and preserve a close and harmonious relationship among its members;
* To work for the common welfare and mutual interest of the members and other personnel of the Parole and Probation Administration and enhance their professional, physical, moral, intellectual, spiritual and cultural growth and socio-economic well-being;
* To determine the relevance and the appropriate role of the Administration personnel in nation-building as changing circumstances warrant and undertake such projects or activities as are necessary or incidental to achieve the purposes and objectives of the League;
* To provide voluntary financial or material assistance to its qualified members and immediate families in case of necessity; and
* To pursue such other activities and endeavours that will ensure the best interest of the League and its members.

The association is national in scope. The PPOLP, Inc. is deemed as the mother or lead organization and under it are local chapters comprising regional personnel associations. There are fifteen local chapters representing Regions I to XII, the National Capital Region, the Cordillera Administrative Region and another distinct chapter for Central Office personnel.

The League has the following executive officers: president, vice-president for Luzon, vice-president for Visayas, vice-president for Mindanao, secretary, treasurer, auditor, public relations officer.

Apart from the executive officers who are elected at large, the local chapters have their respective sets of officers, the presidents of which comprise the Board of Directors of the League. The local chapter officers are elected by personnel within the region.

The PPOLP, Inc. operates through its executive officers, standing committees and local chapter officers. Membership is acquired at local chapter level, so that before one can become a member of the League one must first be a member of a local chapter.

Membership is open to all from the administrator or head of the agency down to the lowest ranked employees provided they hold permanent appointments. There are two categories of members, namely: regular members and honorary members. The former hold posts from chief probation and parole officers down to clerks. Honorary members include the administrator, deputy administrator, regional directors and assistant regional directors.

Every member enjoys the same rights and privileges, the only exception to which is the right to vote and be voted upon which does not apply to honorary members.

Originally, League membership was confined to chief probation and parole officers. The Constitution and By-laws of the League however were amended in 1992 to extend eligibility to all permanent staff regardless of position.

Just over a year after this amendment, membership of all personnel and the affiliation of its fifteen local chapters have yet to be completed. One hundred per cent of all chief probation and parole officers are members.

(Written by Francisco C. Ruivivar, Administrator, Parole and Probation Administration, Department of Justice, the Philippines)

QUALIFICATIONS AND TRAINING

Table 6.2 summarizes the qualifications required of probation officers in each country. Almost all specify a minimum age, and half have a maximum. Seven out of twelve require a professional or technical qualification, and six require a degree. Even in systems where degrees were not required, probation officers often held degrees – with the exception of Papua New Guinea.

Table 6.2 Requirements for becoming a probation officer

	Max. age	Min. age	Prof./ tech. qualific.	Psy. test	Exam	No crim. record	Minimum educational level
New South Wales	No	No	No	No	No	No	No
South Australia	No	Yes	Yes	No	No	No	Degree
Western Australia	Yes	No	Yes	No	No	Yes	High school
Canada	No	Yes	Yes	No	No	No	Degree
Hungary	No	Yes	No	No	No	Yes	Degree
Israel	No	Yes	Yes	No	Yes	No	Degree
Japan	Yes	Yes	No	No	Yes	Yes	No
Papua New Guinea	No	Yes	No	No	No	Yes	High school
The Philippines	Yes	Yes	Yes	Yes	Yes	Yes	Degree
Sweden	No	Yes	Yes	No	No	No	Degree
England and Wales	Yes	Yes	Yes	No	No	No	No
Scotland	Yes	Yes	Yes	No	No	No	No

Notes: The following abbreviations are used in the table: Max. age: maximum age; Min. age: minimum age; Prof./tech. qualific.: professional and/or technical qualification; Psy. test: psychological test; Exam: special exam; No crim. record: no criminal record; High school: high school certificate; Degree: university or college.

Notes:

Australia (New South Wales)
The essentials for new community corrections officers are: ability to assess/counsel/supervise offenders in a community setting, superior self-organizational skills, ability to meet deadlines, well-developed written/oral communication and interpersonal skills, current driver's licence, understanding of multi-cultural issues.

Australia (South Australia)
Whether a criminal record debars an applicant depends on the number and types of offences. Educational requirements are: social work qualifications recognized by the Australian Association of Social Workers, or four-year degree in social work (undergraduate), or two-year post-graduate degree in social work.

Australia (Western Australia)
No minimum age, but is implied by skills/experience. Professional/technical qualification for Level 2/4, but not for Level 2/3. High school certificate for Level 2/3, but university/college degree for Level 2/4.

Canada
The minimum age is 18. The minimum educational requirement is a BA in social science except for Alberta and the North-West Territories which require a diploma and completion of a special examination. The minimum educational requirement for the province of Prince Edward Island is a masters degree.

Japan
Maximum and minimum age limit applies to all government workers; and those with criminal records are debarred from all government employment. Those who want to become probation officers have to pass the national examination for government workers, regardless of their educational background.

Papua New Guinea
Applicants must be of good character and sober habits and have interest in the job. Recruits are generally mature people with considerable experience of life.

Sweden
The entry requirement for probation officers is an academic degree in social work, social or behavioural sciences, law or similar. Appointees usually have several years' experience as social workers or within the correctional service.

United Kingdom (England and Wales)
There is no minimum educational requirement beyond the acquisition of a diploma in social work or equivalent.

United Kingdom (Scotland)
All local authority staff undertaking court reports, probation orders, reports for the Parole Board or mandatory supervision following release from a penal establishment must have a social work qualification – the diploma in social work or equivalent. There is no standard level of qualification for community service officers, those working in supported accommodation facilities or specialist staff offering intensive probation programmes. In practice, staff providing most social work services in the criminal justice system are professionally qualified.

Figure 6.1 shows levels of educational attainment among probation officers in each country. Canada and Scotland are excluded from the figure since no data are available.

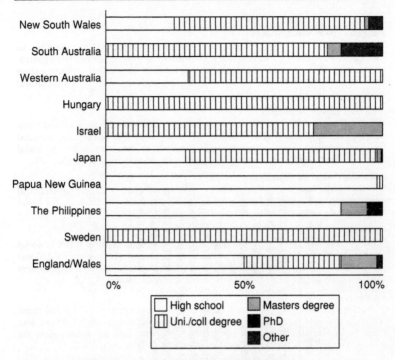

Figure 6.1 Educational level among probation officers

ANNOUNCEMENT OF A JOB VACANCY IN NEW SOUTH WALES (AUSTRALIA)

"Trainee community corrections officer, (2 positions), Dubbo District Office. Pos No: SD 34/92. Total remuneration package valued to $42,568 p.a. (salary $28,418–$37,016). Prepare pre-sentence reports. Supervise offenders released on Community Supervision orders. Provide counselling/assessment of prisoners. *Essential*: Capacity to assess/counsel/supervise offenders in a community setting. Superior self-organisational skills, ability to meet deadlines. Well developed written/oral communication and interpersonal skills. Current driver's licence. Understanding of multi-cultural issues and E.E.O. principles. *Desirable*: Counselling experience, relevant tertiary qualification. *General*: Appointment will be under section 33–34 or 38 of the Public Sector Management Act 1988 pending satisfactory completion of a three-month training course."

Source: Department of Courts Administration (New South Wales, Australia)

Table 6.3 Types of training for probation officers

	Training	Initial	In specific skill	Management
New South Wales	Yes	Compulsory	Not compulsory	Not compulsory
South Australia	Yes	Compulsory	Not compulsory	Not compulsory
Western Australia	Yes	Compulsory	No	Compulsory
Canada	Yes	Compulsory	Compulsory	Not compulsory
Hungary	No	No	No	No
Israel	Yes	No	Compulsory	Compulsory
Japan	Yes	Compulsory	Not compulsory	Not compulsory
Papua New Guinea	Yes	Compulsory	Compulsory	Not compulsory
The Philippines	Yes	Compulsory	Not compulsory	Compulsory
Sweden	Yes	No	Compulsory	Not compulsory
England/Wales	Yes	Compulsory	Compulsory	Not compulsory
Scotland	Yes	Compulsory	Compulsory	Not compulsory

Note: 'Not compulsory' means that there is such training which only selected probation officer can receive; 'No' means that there is no training available.

Table 6.3 summarizes the types of training for probation officers available in each country, and shows whether or not this is compulsory. The term 'initial training' is used to refer both to qualifying training in systems where there is a formal probation qualification, and to induction or preparatory training in systems without formal qualifications. Training in specific skills refers to specialist training aimed at practitioner rather than management grades. All systems except Hungary's provide training of some sort. In most of the countries initial training for newly recruited probation officers is compulsory.

The rest of this section provides a detailed account, country-by-country, of the arrangements for training in each system.

Australia (New South Wales)

Initial training on joining the service is mandatory. The Training and Development Unit of the NSW Probation Service is responsible for this training, which takes three months. The Training and Development Unit is also responsible for additional training in specific skills. Training courses are also provided by other specialist or Government training bodies such as the Centre for Education in Drugs and Alcohol.

The director of the NSW Probation Service is responsible for management training. Only those above field officer level are eligible. There are currently seventy-two officers in management training, which takes eight sessions of a total of sixteen hours' duration over a period of sixteen months. Individual assignments are additional. Management training is not compulsory, but participation is seen as desirable and as a commitment by the officer to developing management skills.

Australia (South Australia)

Tertiary educational institutions are responsible for the initial qualifying training, which takes four years on a full-time basis. There are specialist university training courses for social workers in South Australia, with their own syllabus and textbooks. However, with the move towards a case management/service provision approach to probation work, the Department has been influenced by the American literature on case management and in particular by the British literature on offender development programmes.

Training in specific skills is the responsibility of the Justice Department's Corrections Staff Development Centre. Sixty to seventy per cent of probation officers receive such training in a year. The training, comprising one- or two-day courses, is intended to enhance professional practice rather than help career advancement. The main subjects covered are: group-based programmes; brief intervention; cross-cultural awareness; working with women offenders; working with drug abusing clients; and a monthly 'open forum' for probation officers.

There are other types of training in support of officers' professional development. Paid leave and financial assistance are given to enable probation officers to upgrade their qualifications, to undertake post-graduate training, to attend conferences and seminars and to participate in interstate and overseas officer exchanges.

Management training is again the responsibility of the Corrections Staff Development Centre. Ten per cent of probation officers receive management training in a year, including a two-day introduction to management theory. Justice Department policy is to provide generic training in staff supervision and management for main grade, supervisory and management staff from all occupational streams, i.e. administrative, professional, operational and technical, in order to foster general management skills applicable to and transportable across all streams. Probation officers can attend these courses. Management training is taken into account along with all other factors when officers are being considered for promotion.

Australia (Western Australia)

Initial training is organized by the manager of the Community Corrections Centre where the community corrections officer in question is employed. Its duration may vary. The main subjects covered are: types of orders and procedures associated with them, and office procedures. The training courses are not usually formal, but take the form of individual training for new recruits on a one-to-one basis. Whatever initial training is offered is compulsory.

Thereafter, training in specific skills is provided, covering issues ranging from legislative changes to Aboriginal awareness. Interviewing and counselling skills are expected to have been learnt from studies or experience.

There is management training but on an *ad hoc* basis. This is compulsory when it is offered, and applies to Level 6 and 7 managers. Managers of Community Corrections Centres can approve CCOs' attendance at external management training programmes. There are no figures available concerning the proportion of probation officers who receive management training in a year. The duration of the management training varies. The management training would assist in promotion to positions of manager Level 6 and above.

Canada

The following provinces have training courses for probation officers: Alberta, British Columbia, Ontario and Quebec. In Newfoundland, upon recruitment, new probation officers receive approximately one week of orientation training. The province of Alberta has a Justice Staff College which assists in the completion of centralized probation officer training and managerial training. The training is a combination of on-site supervisor co-ordinated training and central training. A two-week training component for probation officers is compulsory. A wide variety of additional optional training is offered. In general, the department employing the probation officer is responsible for initial training. This tends to be done by the supervisor of the new probation officer, sometimes with help from the provincial headquarters.

Supervisors are generally responsible for providing in-service training for their officers. In Nova Scotia compulsory training for probation officers includes non-violent crisis intervention, occupational health and safety and race relations. There are ongoing professional development opportunities and there is a yearly three-day in-service training programme for all probation officers.

The following course outline from Nova Scotia represents one approach to management training.

MANAGEMENT TRAINING IN NOVA SCOTIA (CANADA)

This box describes the course outline for Nova Scotia's management course. The course comprises a series of workshops, including the following: analysis of the role of the supervisor with a focus upon interpersonal relationships skills, communications, applied human relations, professional attitude and office 'tone setting', team building, conflict and conflict resolution strategies, leadership and leadership training, identifying problem areas and taking leadership roles in problem solving, and the role of the supervisor with respect to the management of the organization.

Technical Aspects of Supervision

Training addresses the acts and statutes both federally and provincially which impact on the supervisor's role in the criminal justice system of Nova Scotia, and identifies the principles, mission, goals and objectives of the criminal justice system, the Ministry of the Solicitor-General, the correctional services, the organizational structure of criminal justice and the Solicitor-General's Department of Nova Scotia. It also covers contemporary issues such as racism, sexism, affirmative action programmes, equality in the application of programmes (i.e. the ability to pay fines versus non-ability to pay fines in the fine option programme), including conflict of interests, moral, ethical issues and systems to monitor potential problem areas.

Performance appraisal

The main elements of performance appraisal includes workload planning, coaching and monitoring and the performance appraisal interview. These concepts are built into the process school of management. Priority is placed on: frequent review of problems and issues; performance appraisal; coaching of staff to improve performance; and ensuring that they understand the relationships between strategic planning, tactical planning, organizational policy, and evaluation.

The administration of collective agreements

Addresses how managers must work within collective agreements, identifies the relationship of collective agreements to regulations and legislation, and to policy and procedures.

Approaches to problem solving are discussed within the collective agreement, together with staff discipline, the grievance procedure, and problem identification and remedies.

Administrative report writing

Addresses reports which are generally prepared for supervisors on incidents, planning reports, evaluation reports, etc. Report writing and style, contents and confidentiality of reports are discussed.

Workload management

Addresses workloads and workload management planning. Identifies strategies and approaches for dealing with workloads and using time efficiently.

Interviewing and investigating

Includes strategies for conducting interviews which are mainly fact finding in determining what has taken place in various situations or incidents. Pre-planning, undertaking and critiquing interviews are discussed. The relationship to interviewing, interrogation and statement taking in the criminal process is clarified. Managing conflict. Managing diversity, personnel selection techniques.

The management of crisis

This course addresses the concept of crisis from the perspective of public welfare issues, public order issues, individual crises and group conflict crises. The states of crisis are discussed and organizational responses in the various stages are clarified. The need for contingency planning is accented with discussion focusing upon cross-organization relationships in addressing crisis, and the potential crisis management team.

Stress management and lifestyles for supervisors/ managers

Course includes clarification of the concept of stress and the need for understanding lifestyles which contribute to healthy positive staff members. Strategies of approach to dealing with stress and stress management are discussed.

Critical incident stress for supervisors/managers

This course will address critical incidents and the impact they have on human beings in cognitive, affective and behavioural perspectives. Interventions for dealing with critical incident stress, operational debriefs and critical incident stress debriefs are discussed as part of this programme.

(Information provided by Gordon Parry, Co-ordinator Sentencing Team, Department of Justice, Canada)

Hungary

There is no training available for probation officers at present, but it is intended to organize a special post-graduate course based in law faculties with the collaboration of other faculties. It is planned to establish a special examination along the lines of those relating to sentencing, prosecution and advocacy.

Israel

University social work schools are responsible for initial training.

In order to meet the constantly changing needs of its target population, the Juvenile Probation Service has developed a multi-faceted programme of in-service training for its personnel. The techniques of supervision and monitoring employed by the Service are integrally linked with a system of individualized programmes that include counselling and specialized instruction, as well as professional supervision.

Management training is compulsory for district probation officers. The Director of the Service and the Ministry In-Service Training Department are responsible for management training. About 20 per cent of probation officers receive management training in a year. The management training takes six months, and the main subjects covered are: management techniques; introduction to the sociology of Israel; introduction to economics and statistics; computer technology.

Japan

The Research and Training Institute of the Ministry of Justice is responsible for training probation officers, in close consultation with the Rehabilitation Bureau of the Ministry of Justice. The Institute runs a variety of courses on a regular basis.

Initial training is in three stages: fifty days training at the Research and Training Institute; then about six months on-the-job training at the probation office to which the probation officer belongs; and finally, thirty days further training at the Research and Training Institute. Initial training thus takes about nine months in total. The main subjects covered are: probation laws, regulations and procedures; parole, aftercare and pardons; law and legal procedures; criminology; behavioural sciences; counselling, casework and related fields; case studies; introduction of the function of relevant agencies; liberal arts; fieldwork. The Research and Training Institute of the Ministry of Justice publishes a textbook on the Japanese rehabilitation system.

Some seventy probation officers a year receive in-service training in specific professional skills, on one of three annual courses run by the Research and Training Institute. The courses last thirty-five, twenty and fifteen days respectively. The training is considered important for career advancement. The main subjects covered are: probation laws, regulations and procedures; parole, aftercare and pardons; behavioural sciences; counselling, casework and related fields; and fieldwork.

There are two types of management training courses for different levels of officers. The course for top managers – newly appointed directors of probation offices – is virtually compulsory, but that for middle managers is not. (Middle managers are chiefs of the various sections of the Probation Office or the Parole Board.) In general, ten top managers receive management training annually, attending a five-day course; and twenty middle managers attend a twelve-day course. The main subjects covered by the courses are: probation laws, regulations and procedures of probation; parole, aftercare and pardons; administration and staff management.

Papua New Guinea

The last three years have seen the Probation Service developing its own training policy for in-house and external training. A training programme has been developed with specific course modules to train officers in the skills required for various aspects of the job. External training courses have also been identified and officers who qualify are sent on them. The in-house training courses are delivered very largely by experienced staff in the Training Section of the Probation Service; but outsiders are also brought in from time to time.

The Training Section is responsible for initial training, which takes six weeks. The main subjects covered are: history of PNG Probation Service, the Probation Act and the role of probation officers, the court system in PNG, ways of sentencing, court work programmes, pre-sentence reports, interviewing and counselling skills, and supervision of offenders. Training has been developed to reflect the needs of PNG.

The Training Section is also responsible for in-service training in specific skills. Almost all probation officers attend at least one training course each year. Courses usually last between three days and a week. (Though the induction course for new officers lasts six weeks, counselling is one week, case management one week, Parole Act one week, pre-sentence reports one week and criminal compensation one week.) This training is considered important for career advancement.

In relation to management training, it is the responsibility of the chief probation officer to ensure all management staff are appropriately trained. Management skills are not normally taught in induction courses. Whilst officers in charge of provincial or major offices are given in-house management training courses of one week, senior staff do attend relevant management courses at the government's Public Service Training Institute which is a responsibility of the Personnel Management Department. The CPO recommends officers for the courses, and the Secretary of the Attorney-General's Department makes the final decision. The proportion of probation officers receiving management training in a year depends on the number of management positions to be filled. Management training at the Institute lasts from six weeks to nine months, depending on the type of course. Institute courses which are considered relevant to

Probation Service management include: report writing and communication skills; skills in working with people; management skills; and financial management. Staff evaluation procedures carried out twice a year also identify training needs of individual officers, and appropriate training is then provided.

Training in specific skills is done on a needs basis; some courses are compulsory, specially those concerned with the implementation of new programmes, policy changes and new laws.

The Philippines

The Training Division of the Parole and Probation Administration is responsible for the in-house training of all probation officers, in both basic and specialized courses.

For initial training, all newly appointed probation officers are required to undergo the Probation Officer Basic Course; all other employees are required to attend the Employee Orientation Course. The initial probation officer training takes one month. There are no formally adopted textbooks but reading materials gathered from various sources covering laws, rules and administrative guidance have been compiled and are regularly updated.

The Training Division has primary responsibility for in-service training to provide specific professional skills. Training courses are largely conducted in-house; where governmental or other agencies offer specialized training programmes which are of value to probation work, selected staff may be authorized to enrol in programmes with tuition paid by the Parole and Probation Administration. All supervising parole and probation officers underwent training in the Indeterminate Sentence Law in 1990 when the supervision of parolees was transferred to the Parole and Probation Administration. Selected chief probation and parole officers (CPPOs) and senior probation and parole officers (SPPOs) were required to attend seminar workshops on pre-parole investigation and parole report writing in 1991 when the pre-parole investigation function was assigned to the Parole and Probation Administration (PPA) by the Board of Pardons and Parole. Ninety per cent of the CPPOs and 30 per cent of SPPOs attended the training course. Training courses in specific skills generally take one to two weeks. The training is considered important for career advancement as it upgrades the skills of employees, increases their efficiency and effectiveness, increases their contribution to the productivity of the organization, and hence prospects for promotion.

A government-wide management training programme is provided by the Career Executive Service Board and is required for all government officials including the PPA as a prerequisite for appointment to positions in the Career Executive Service, the highest level in the Civil Service. Positions of administrator, assistant administrator, regional and assistant regional director of the PPA belong to the Career Executive Service. The Parole and Probation Administration through its Training Division, gives a two-week Basic Supervisory Development Course for chief probation and parole officers. All chief probation and parole officers who have not attended such a course and supervising probation officers who have been promoted to CPPO receive management training. The duration of the management training is ten days. Officers who complete the course have a decided advantage over those who have not in terms of consideration for promotion to higher positions. However, since the training is compulsory, eventually all CPPOs finish the course.

Sweden

Many probation officers have their first contact with probation work as trainees (serving internships) during their academic studies at the School of Social Work. Other university departments also provide training which mixes theory with one or two practical training periods.

Probation officers are usually required to hold a relevant degree (in social work, for example, social or behavioural sciences or law), as well as several years' work experience in a related field; thus they will already have received some relevant training. There is no initial training specifically for probation officers at present, though the staff training department is currently considering basic training for new recruits.

In-service training in specific skills is provided through locally and regionally organized courses of varying lengths. University courses on subjects relevant to probation work are mounted from time to time by universities in collaboration with the regional authorities. Training in specific skills received is considered important for career advancement.

The National Prison and Probation Administration is responsible for management training. Ten per cent of probation officers receive management training of some sort each year. Training to prepare staff for chief probation officer posts takes two years. Other courses are much shorter, lasting between a day and a week. Management training, which focuses on human resource management, has a great impact on career advancement.

United Kingdom (England and Wales)

Initial or qualifying training takes two years, and is provided by universities and colleges, in partnership with probation and social work agencies – though theses arrangements are now under review. Students completing courses receive a Diploma in Social Work. This qualification (or a recognized equivalent) is a statutory requirement for probation officers. The courses are competence based, in that they are validated according to their ability to equip students with specified competences. The courses aim to equip students with generalist social work skills, which may be supplemented by a specialism, one of which is probation work. Some thirty courses run probation 'options' which are recognized by the Home Office. Courses cover social work and probation theory and practice, supplemented by practical experience through placements in probation or social work departments. Up to three placements are sandwiched between study on the course.

Responsibility for ensuring proper provision of in-service training lies with the chief probation officer of each area. Specific skills should be taught in pre-qualifying training, but officers often need refresher training or have to acquire new professional skills. Courses are run (or purchased) by probation areas, or by Regional Staff Development Units (which are being reorganized into a national system by the Home Office Probation Training Unit). For example, all main-grade officers and senior probation officers were given training in 1992 on the 1991 Criminal Justice Act. The duration of the training in specific skills varies. In-service training in specific skills received is considered important for career advancement. Some of this training is compulsory or near-compulsory – e.g. training on certain new legislation: some is heavily recommended.

Responsibility for ensuring proper provision of management training again lies with the chief probation officer of each area.

Management skills are not taught in pre-qualifying training; courses are run (or purchased) by probation areas, or by Regional Staff Development Units. Some management training for senior managers is provided or supported directly by the Home Office. Management training is not a prerequisite for promotion to senior probation officer, though some areas run courses for probation officers who are applying for SPO posts. Promotion thereafter would be hindered by lack of training. Though management training is not generally compulsory, it is obviously advisable for anyone seeking promotion to management grades.

In-service training, whether on specific professional skills or on management, is also provided by a number of academic institutions within a framework of continuing professional training established by the CCETSW (Central Council for Education and Training in Social Work). It uses credit accumulation and transfer and comprises two levels of attainment – a post-qualifying award and an advanced award – along four routes: practice, management, research and training.

United Kingdom (Scotland)

Pre-qualifying or initial training for social work staff carrying equivalent responsibilities to probation officers in England and Wales takes the form of a course resulting in a Diploma of Social Work – the same qualification that is required of probation officers in England and Wales. Courses last two years and are either free-standing or included in a three- or four-year degree course such as a BA in Social Policy and Social Work. They are concerned with general skills in social work practice, but some include skills specific to criminal justice work. Students undertake agency-based work which is supported by skills training in the university and by accredited agency-based student supervisors (eighty day placements in 'an area of particular practice', e.g. criminal justice work, during the second year of the course).

In-service training is the responsibility of individual local authorities, supplemented by training initiatives financed by central government. A programme of advanced studies in criminal justice was established in Scotland in 1993 within the framework for post-qualifying training established by the CCETSW (see entry for England and Wales). It is funded by the Scottish Office and involves two years' part-time study, including one year of monitoring practice in the agency setting. It offers a twin track programme of advanced practice and management. It is actively supported by local authorities and the take-up rate has been good – sixteen students in its first year, all of whom are criminal justice practitioners.

The duration of the training in specific skills varies considerably. Induction programmes tend to last about three days. In-service training courses can last from half a day to five days. In time, it is expected that many of these in-service training programmes will be able to submit themselves for validation with a view to contributing to a post-qualifying award (credit accumulation). Training in specific skills is considered important for career advancement. Available evidence suggests everyone coming off post-qualifying certificated offender programmes is achieving career advancement either into management or into academic posts. The main subjects covered are: induction; duties and responsibilities of practitioners; groupwork methods; assessment (use of risk of custody scales); confronting offending behaviour; new legislation and associated national standards and guidance; management practice; project development; working with particular types of offenders and offences (for example, sex offenders, violence, alcohol and drugs); monitoring and evaluation techniques; service planning.

Responsibility for management training again lies with the local authority in each area. Management skills are not taught in qualifying training courses. Some in-house management training is provided but the bulk of it is purchased from a range of training bodies. In 1992, the Scottish Office sponsored the Institute of Management to run nine courses in initial management training for recent entrants to first line management posts in criminal justice services: there were ninety participants. These courses are continuing. Three academic institutions in Scotland run post-qualifying courses in social work management, all of which are currently being used by local authorities for staff working in the criminal justice field – all lead to a masters degree. Current estimates suggest that approximately twenty-three local authority criminal justice workers are participating in post-qualifying courses leading to an advanced qualification in management such as a masters degree. Ninety staff participated in initial management training in 1993. All senior and middle managers providing criminal justice services undertook a two-day training programme in strategic planning of criminal justice services in 1993. Post-qualifying training courses leading to the advanced award are two year, usually part-time. Others are usually quite short, on average two or three days. The management training is not a prerequisite for promotion to management posts at present but the tendency is in that direction, especially for middle/senior managers providing criminal justice services. Increasing numbers of staff are taking up management training opportunities and an increasing number of management staff already have management training experience.

SALARIES OF PROBATION OFFICERS

Figure 6.2 presents information on absolute levels of pay, expressed in US dollars. Given how widely the cost of living varies in the countries included in the study, it is difficult to interpret differences in levels of pay, of course. However, probation officers in most of the countries belonging to the former Commonwealth receive broadly similar salaries. Japan pays its probation officers the highest salaries – but also has a high cost of living. Probation

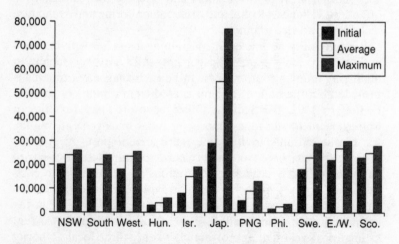

Figure 6.2 Initial, average and maximum salary of probation officers

Note: The following abbreviations are used in the figure: NSW: New South Wales; South: South Australia; West.: Western Australia; Hun.: Hungary; Isr.: Israel; Jap.: Japan; PNG: Papua New Guinea; Phi.: the Philippines; Swe.: Sweden; E./W.: England and Wales; Sco.: Scotland. The salaries are calculated in US dollars per year.

Table 6.4 Comparison of salary with other occupations

	1	2	3	4	5
New South Wales	PO	Teacher	Nurse	Police	Nat. wage
South Australia	PO	Teacher	Nurse	Police	—
Western Australia	Police	PO	Nurse	Teacher	Nat. wage
Hungary	Police	PO	Teacher	Nat. wage	Nurse
Israel	Teacher	Police	PO	Nurse	Nat. wage
Japan	Police	Teacher	PO	Nat. wage	Nurse
Papua New Guinea	PO	Teacher	Police	Nurse	Nat. wage
The Philippines	PO	Teacher	Police	Nurse	Nat. wage
Sweden	Police	Teacher	PO	Nurse	Nat. wage
England and Wales	Police	PO	Nat. wage	Teacher	Nurse
Scotland	Police	PO	Nat. wage	Teacher	Nurse

Note: This table shows the comparison between the salaries of probation officers and other professions on the initial level in each country (1-5 refers to the rank in order, 1 being the highest). The following abbreviations are used in the table: Nat. wage: national male industrial wage; Nurse: nurse in public hospital; Police: police officer; PO: probation officer; Teacher: teacher in state school.

officers in developing countries generally receive relatively low salaries.

Table 6.4 compares probation salaries with other professions. Information was not available for Canada. In six of the eleven other probation systems probation officers are paid more than police officers; in seven they are paid more than teachers; in all systems they get more than the national average and more than nurses.

CAREER ADVANCEMENT

Career advancement is not a simple matter to research. Countries will vary in the weight they attach to formal academic and professional qualifications, for example, and to length and breadth of experience. At one extreme some countries have very precise criteria relating to time in post, level of qualifications and so on; and at the other extreme, judgements are more subjective and based on evaluation of performance in the job. From the information at our disposal we are unable to distinguish effectively between formality of selection procedures and formality of selection criteria. Countries have combined the subjective and the formal in a variety of ways, and it is hard to see any obvious trends or patterns, except that Commonwealth countries seem to be less formal than others. In Figure 6.3 each country has been placed on a five-point scale, where a score of 1 reflects very formal requirements and a score of 5 reflects an absence of formal requirements. Each system was scored on the scale by the relevant country expert.

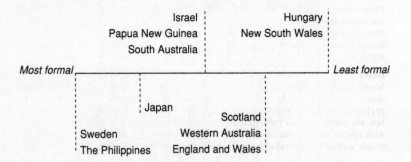

Figure 6.3 Formality of promotion among probation officers

Notes:

Australia (New South Wales)
Selection criteria include: ability to work and manage within the Probation Service's mission statement; to effectively manage resources and Service programmes; demonstrated high level ability in achieving outcomes which optimize Service objectives; highly developed communication and analytical skills are significant.

Australia (South Australia)
Although in probation and parole the emphasis is on professional social work as the basis for intervention with clients, career promotion currently is only possible via the staff supervisory/managerial avenue, thus limiting the development of professional expertise beyond basic grade level. The restructuring of the Department, resulting in a flatter structure and rationalization of functions and low staff turnover has significantly reduced promotion opportunities. Because of these limitations, an ability to identify with and advance the goals of the Department as well as create harmonious relationships with colleagues and superiors are important factors in securing promotion.

Australia (Western Australia)
Attention is paid to the extent to which individuals have sought to broaden their knowledge of contemporary issues relevant to management and policy within the broader public service, not just within their own work area.

Canada
Most probation officer positions are filled via regular public service entry requirements. Promotion within the service is done in accordance with the public service requirements in that province. In general, each position has a job description which is classified for salary purposes. There are basic requirements including knowledge/education, experience and personal suitability. Jobs are advertised, and selection usually made through interviews. Candidates are assessed against the required qualifications on the basis of the interview, checks of references and work performance. The job is offered to the candidate who ranks first among the applicants after the selection process. One province has stated that the most important, over-riding quality for promotion is demonstrated commonsense. Although this quality is the most difficult to measure, it over-rides experience and educational level.

Hungary
A college or university degree is required. There is no official promotion system. Promotion to management level depends on the decision of the president of the relevant county court. The president's decision takes into account the professional qualification, the length of experience, relationship with colleagues and fitness of that probation officer. The first and the last requirements are the most important.

Israel
Senior posts are filled by an evaluation committee, which requires that all candidates have at least seven years' experience in social work or management; preference is given to candidates with an MA degree. The following characteristics are considered to be essential to career promotion: ability to communicate with clients, therapeutic ability, organizational ability, a good relationship with the courts and other relevant agencies in the community.

Japan
Although casework ability and social resource management ability are necessary for becoming a good probation officer, management ability, to pursue organizational

goals, to get along with colleagues and to give training and material and spiritual support to young officers, are also important for career promotion.

Papua New Guinea
Commitment to the job and willingness to 'go the extra mile' is an indication the officer believes in the work he/she is doing towards improving the criminal justice system. Where opportunities exist these officers can expect quick promotion. The single most important factor influencing career promotion is availability of staff accommodation (housing) in a particular location. Given that the probation system has been only recently been set up, experience amongst probation officers is very limited.

The Philippines
The following characteristics are considered to be important to career promotion: commitment to the goals of probation and a genuine desire to help clients who have personal, adjustment and legal problems; ability to relate to colleagues, superiors and subordinates, and to work with a team; ability to network with other government agencies and establish linkages with community agencies and elicit public participation in the probation programme.

Sweden
The standard work of the probation service is maintained in the first place through a high level of required qualifications. The prerequisite for chief, assistant chief and ordinary probation officers is an academic degree. Appointees usually have several years' counselling experience in the correctional service, with a local social welfare authority or in institutional care. Whereas formal qualifications were earlier emphasized, personal ability is now regarded as equally important. As the professional qualifications of a probation officer are the same as those for several other professions within the social and administrative field, it is possible to advance one's career without staying in the probation service.

United Kingdom (England and Wales)
Promotion is generally through open competition for advertised jobs, and selection is via a formal interview process. One important factor must be the ability to pursue and advance the goals of the organization. As there is a degree of conflict within the organization about these goals, it is to be expected that those who are hostile to the evolving policy of their area will limit their promotion chances.

United Kingdom (Scotland)
The following characteristics are considered to be important for career promotion: commitment to the service – its objectives and professional standards – and to the agency providing the service; the capacity to advance the quality of service within the opportunities and constraints of the agency setting; confidence in one's professional identity as a social worker and in one's skills as a practitioner; leadership qualities such as human resource management skills; an understanding of the service in relation both to the agency and to the community it serves; and the ability to work in multi-disciplinary and multi-agency settings.

Chapter 7

Variations in probation function

Mike Hough

This chapter examines variations in function between the probation systems covered by the study. By way of introduction, it considers the range of functions covered by each system. The core of the chapter examines how different systems approach the core task of providing probation supervision. (The term is used here in a very inclusive sense, to embrace not only counselling but surveillance, and activities with a reparative function.) Finally, the chapter discusses the question of role conflict – the tensions between care and control – which can emerge in some probation systems.

THE RANGE OF PROBATION FUNCTIONS

All the probation systems included by definition some form of probation supervision either as a substitute for a court sentence or as a sentence in its own right. Most performed a wide range of additional functions, summarized in Table 7.1.

Pre-trial

One of the clearest points to emerge from the table is that at the time of the study, all systems with the exception of Japan and the Philippines provided the courts with some form of pre-trial report on offenders. Japan follows the very clear principle that the role of the probation service starts only after sentence. In the Philippines, post-sentence investigations are carried out only after a sentence of imprisonment has been passed, to help the court decide whether or not to suspend sentence; the reports are thus functionally the equivalent of pre-trial reports elsewhere. In other

Table 7.1 Functions at different stages of the criminal justice process

	Aul. NSW	Sth	West.	Can.	Hun.	Isr.	Jap.	PNG	Phi.	Swe.	UK E./W.	Sco.
Probation supervision	X	X	X	X	X	X	X	X	X	X	X	X
Pre-trial												
Social enquiry report	X	X	X	X	X	X	X	X	X	X	X	X
Pre-bail assessment	X	X				X					X	X
Bail supervision	X		X	X								
Pre-trial counselling								X				
During custody												
Pre-release assessment		X		X		X	X		X	X	X	
Preparation for release		X	X		X	X	X			X		X
Post-release												
Supervision of offenders after release	X	X	X				X			X	X	

Note: The following abbreviations are used in the table: Aul.: Australia; NSW: New South Wales; Sth: South Australia; West.: Western Australia; Can.: Canada; Hun.: Hungary; Isr.: Israel; Jap.: Japan; PNG: Papua New Guinea; Phi.: the Philippines; Swe.: Sweden; UK: United Kingdom; E./W.: England/Wales; Sco.: Scotland.

words, probation officers in almost all the systems we examined can exercise some control over the process whereby offenders are selected for probation. Indeed the practice of preparing reports focusing on non-legal variables (about the offender's background and circumstances) is consistent with the concept of 'special selection' in the 1951 UN definition of probation discussed at the start of Chapter 1.

Other forms of pre-trial work were less widespread, but some countries were extending their pre-trial role. Five systems provided some form of pre-bail assessment, and four provided some form of supervision or support of bailees. Though other systems undoubtedly provide offenders with informal advice and information before trial, the Papua New Guinea expert alone identified this as a significant function.

During custody (throughcare)

The study paid little attention to the work of probation officers with offenders whilst in prison or after release. It is clear, however, that nine out of the twelve systems undertook work of some sort with prisoners – in the form either of pre-release assessment (e.g. for parole), or of work preparing offenders for release. Administrative arrangements were very varied. In some systems, such as New South Wales, no such work was done simply because the function was performed by a separate parole service. In some, probation officers – or social workers – were seconded full-time to prisons. Notably, England and Wales had about a tenth of its probation officers seconded to the Prison Service; similar work was done in South Australia and Scotland by social workers. Elsewhere, throughcare work was undertaken solely by field probation officers.

Post-release (aftercare)

Table 7.1 shows that all systems covered by the study undertake supervision of offenders on release from prison, with the exception of Canada where this work is done by the – organizationally separate – Parole Service. In most cases this takes the form of parole supervision. As with pre-trial functions, the role of probation in supervising offenders on release from custody seems to be developing in many systems, with new or substantially revised systems of parole/early release, generally involving mandatory supervision, in Australia, Papua New Guinea, the Philippines and the United Kingdom.

Division of time between functions

Figure 7.1 shows the proportion of time devoted to different tasks in each system except Hungary's and Israel's, for which no information was available. Different methodologies have been used in different countries, ranging from large-scale workload surveys in England and Wales and Canada, for example, to the best guesses and professional judgement of the experts or probation officers co-opted by them. Different definitions have also been used for the various categories; for example, Sweden and England and Wales include management of their volunteers within the 'supervision' category. Definitions of 'administration' are certainly not consistent: there is no reason to conclude from the Figure that the administrative burden on Japanese probation officers is six times that of British ones. The explanation is that the latter's figures have not distinguished between core functions and the administrative work generated by these functions. Despite its limitations, we have included the Figure as it provides 'order of magnitude' estimates of the breakdown of probation workloads in different countries.

PROBATION SUPERVISION

Our questionnaire devoted a fair amount of space to the way in which probation supervision was carried out, and the experts' returns provided a great deal of valuable information. This section aims to identify the key dimensions on which systems varied, drawing on the expert reports to illustrate differences and similarities.

Dimension 1: from therapy to punishment

As was discussed in Chapter 1, two key elements of probation as it emerged at the end of the nineteenth and the start of the twentieth centuries were the conditional suspension of punishment and the supervision of offenders, involving some form of guidance or treatment. Several of the systems which we examined were in

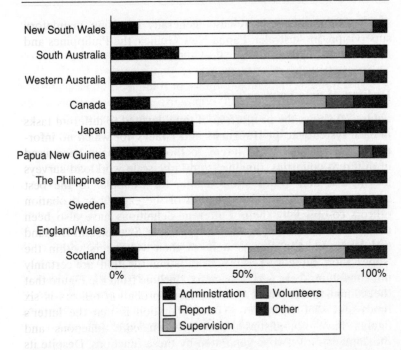

Figure 7.1 Task proportion of probation officers

Note: The following abbreviations are used in the figure: administration (administrative work, other than report writing; preparing and updating probationers' file); reports (preparing court reports); supervision (supervision of individual probationers); volunteers (management of volunteer workers); other (involvement in group activities, union, association; non-probation-related work, such as certain duties related to divorce; liaison with other agencies).

a process of evolution or transition, whereby the suspensive nature of probation was being reduced and the functions of probation supervision were being broadened to include more unambiguously penal functions such as reparation, compensation and straightforward restriction of liberty. This trend can be understood partly as a pragmatic response to the pressure on prison systems caused by rising crime – the more the emphasis on the suspension of punishment and on the therapeutic aims of probation, the less it can do service as a convincing alternative to imprisonment for offenders who have committed crimes which fall in the middle range of severity. The shift can also be understood as one of the consequences of the revival of interest in deserts-based penological theories; the more suspensive the nature of probation, the less it can be accommodated in a sentencing framework which stresses proportionality.

All of our systems retained at their core a form of probation supervision which was recognizably that identified by the 1951 UN definition as involving guidance or treatment. Those countries which made extensive use of volunteer supervisors, notably Japan and Sweden, not surprisingly approached supervision less as a technological treatment and more as an exercise in common-sense; lay supervisors aimed to provide a mix of advice, moral encouragement and practical help. In Israel, the counselling function retained a psychotherapeutic or clinical vocabulary; the extent to which this was reflected in practice is unclear. The 'cognitive-behavioural' approach seemed well established in the United Kingdom and Old Commonwealth countries (McGuire and Priestley 1985; Ross and Fabiano 1985; Ross et al. 1988). Grounded in social learning theory, the approach has a lot in common with the sort of intuitive approach that a lay counsellor might adopt, combining moral persuasion with practical support and skills; what marks it apart from both commonsense counselling and more clinical approaches is its structured approach, and its use of groupwork. It places emphasis on:

- getting the offender to confront his/her offending and recognize the harm he/she does;
- identifying the factors which underlie offending and getting the offender to recognize these;
- teaching the offender new skills to avoid the circumstances which lead to offending; and
- providing material help towards the same end.

The extent to which counselling (of whatever brand) formed the *central* function was obviously hard for us to judge, but in some countries it clearly was. Thus the experts for Hungary, Israel, Japan and Scotland all made reference to counselling or casework as the foundation of probation, and it was clear from their accounts that the suspensive character of probation remained fairly intact. The experts for these countries made the point that providing counselling and other forms of social work help inevitably involves a degree of monitoring and control, if only to ensure that offenders actually observed the conditions of their order; leaving this aside, however, control and surveillance were not construed as punitive or correctional in purpose.

Sweden and England and Wales provide examples of systems in transition. In both, counselling or casework remained a central, if not dominant, mode of operation; but in both, probation is now a sentence in its own right. This occurred in England and Wales as part of a package of legislative changes – contained in the 1991 Criminal Justice Act – intended to incorporate community penalties into a coherent deserts-based sentencing framework. The probation service in England and Wales is also responsible for the administration of – essentially reparative – community service orders, though significantly, the supervision of offenders serving CSOs is carried out by non-professionals rather than by qualified staff. At the time of fieldwork, both Sweden and England and Wales were planning experimental or pilot forms of electronic monitoring. (In England and Wales, however, the role of the probation service in this is likely to be marginal.)

The other systems in the study had more of a 'mixed economy', where functions other than counselling or casework had a more central role, with a much more explicit recognition of penal or correctionalist objectives. Amongst the industrially developed countries, Australia provided the clearest examples. All three of the Australian states in the study emphasized that casework and surveillance are integral components of case management, and that social work intervention was provided only as and when appropriate. Western Australia substantially reorganized its probation system in 1989, replacing a 'welfare' model of probation with a 'justice' one; the correctional aspirations of the system were stated unambiguously in the new title for probation officers, community corrections officers. Elsewhere, Papua New Guinea and the Philippines also showed considerable eclecticism in the elements that were built into probation supervision: orders could include community work, compensation, reparation or (occasionally) forms of curfew.

Dimension 2: bureaucrat or professional?

Many of the systems displayed characteristics both of bureaucracies and of the professions, and none had all the hallmarks of traditional professions. However, it can be seen from Chapter 6 that probation officers in some of the better established systems could lay claim to professional status in terms of the autonomy of their working practices, for example, their entry qualifications and the existence of professional associations. (Where systems had professional associations, however, these seemed often to operate less as mechanisms for self-regulation than as trades unions.) Israel and Scotland probably provide the clearest examples of professionalization; Hungary and Papua New Guinea lie at the other end of the spectrum.

One might have predicted that there would be a close correlation between systems where 'casework was king' and those with clear profession status – and that a 'correctionalist' emphasis might be associated with more bureaucratic or managerialist systems. The latter seemed true but the former not. Casework occupied a central position in some of the more unequivocally bureaucratic systems. Thus in both Sweden and Japan there was no requirement for any professional probation qualification; the emphasis in training was on induction courses; and probation officers were central government civil servants in both systems. Yet in both systems the counselling function was clearly the dominant one. (Significantly, both systems used volunteers as well as professionals to supervise offenders, as is discussed below.)

Although our evidence is tentative, shifting the focus of probation from counselling to correctionalism seems unlikely to be readily achieved in systems with a well-established base of therapeutic professionalism. It is noteworthy that in England and Wales central government efforts to shift the balance of probation work away from counselling towards forms of supervision with a more explicitly punitive element have met with strong resistance from the professionally qualified staff. Arguably the system is able to deliver both rehabilitative and reparative forms of community penalty only by virtue of a clear organizational distinction between professionally qualified probation officers and the largely unqualified community service staff.

Dimension 3: the use of community resources

There were very marked differences in the extent to which systems exploited community resources; and amongst countries which did so there were significant variations in the form which this took. There were two main variants, which were not mutually exclusive: bringing volunteers into the organization, to supervise offenders under the oversight of probation officers; and drawing on community facilities outside the probation system.

The use of volunteers is considered in detail in the next chapter. To anticipate the main points to emerge, all except New South Wales, Hungary and Israel made use of volunteers. Three systems made substantial use of volunteers: Japan's system is built around volunteers, who supervise the majority of offenders on probation; almost half of Swedish probationers are supervised by lay supervisors; and the aim in Papua New Guinea is that volunteers should supervise the majority of minor offenders, leaving the smaller number of serious cases to probation officers. Volunteers elsewhere generally had a role in supervising offenders, usually under the direction of a probation officer. The Hungarian system until recently made use of supervision by offenders' colleagues in the workplace, though this practice has had to be suspended, at least temporarily, in the face of the economic difficulties and high unemployment currently faced there. The use of volunteers in the United Kingdom seemed relatively limited, especially in relation to supervision. It is plausible that systems which are heavily professionalized, as in England and Wales and in Israel, are less able than others to develop the role of volunteers creatively.

The attractiveness of volunteers lies partly in the very fact that they are a near-free resource; but it is noteworthy that the two countries in our study which made greatest use of volunteers – Japan and Sweden – were amongst the wealthiest. Their use of volunteers was motivated less by considerations of economy than by the idea that reintegrating offenders into the community can be most effectively achieved by that community.

The other main way in which community resources were exploited was in drawing on facilities outside the probation system. This seemed to be a significant and growing feature of most of the systems we looked at. In several systems, the role of probation officers was explicitly that of case manager rather than case worker. Their work was variously described as negotiating access to services (South Australia), acting as brokers of services (Canada), a bridge between the needs of probationers and the resources available in the community (the Philippines), working as intermediaries between the offender and relevant agencies (Sweden) and as social resource managers (Scotland).

Several factors seem to underlie this. In some countries,

especially those with well-resourced social services, the role of probation officer as broker to social services has been long established. One of the fundamental principles of the Swedish system, for example, is that of 'normalization' whereby offenders detained for correctional treatment have the same rights as others to society's resources for care and support. More recently in developed countries, pressures for improvements in public sector efficiency have resulted in the 'out-sourcing' (to use current managerialist jargon) of specialist functions, such as services for drug abusers. Our experts from less affluent countries stressed lack of probation resources as a key factor in mobilizing community support and facilities; in Hungary, social resource management was seen as the most desirable mode of probation supervision, but the current dislocation of the economy made it very hard to locate any exploitable community resources.

Behind these justifications often lay a more persuasive rationale, which was that community resources were uniquely appropriate to attempts to reintegrate offenders into society. Scotland's Statement of Principles for Social Work Services in the Criminal Justice System sets this out well:

> Local authorities cannot fully comply with their responsibilities within the criminal justice system without the confidence, support and assistance not just of the judiciary and criminal justice agencies but also of the wider community.

SOCIAL RESOURCE MANAGEMENT IN THE PHILIPPINES

Other than the use of volunteers, the probation service establishes and maintains links with government organizations (GOs) and non-governmental organizations (NGOs). These include agencies involved in manpower and skills development, employment, youth welfare, health care, education and family welfare. Included as part of the network are religious organizations, professional associations (doctors, lawyers, etc.), hospitals, educational institutions and social services within the community.

By networking with these agencies, the probation offices are able to provide their clients with programmes and services needed for their rehabilitation and at the same time imbue them with a sense of nationhood and civic consciousness, to wit:

1   Programmes geared toward national development goals:

- forest conservation. Offenders convicted of *Kaingin* (slash-and-burn) farming are retrained and thereafter allowed to participate in social forestry contracts (reforestation and tree farming) and given government subsidy and compensation for their work;

- marine conservation. Offenders convicted of illegal fishing (explosives or poison) or destruction of corals are retrained and given start-up money for purchase/lease of fishing boats and gear through livelihood assistance loans;

- loan assistance programmes. Non-profit corporations or foundations as well as government agencies and financial institutions tasked with the development of small and medium-scale industries assist probationers engaged in entrepreneurial enterprises by providing them with loans or start-up money for such activities as RTW garments manufacture, handicraft making, food processing and preservation, machine/radio/electrical shop operations and other cottage industries.

2   Programmes geared towards local community development activities:

- probationers and parolees are allowed to participate in town or village activities as volunteer fire or traffic aides, crime or drug-watch volunteers and other activities directed towards the maintenance of law and order in the community;

- group activities such as tree-planting along the highways, cleanliness, sanitation and beautification of public buildings and parks.

3   Programmes geared towards client empowerment, self-reliance and personal growth:

- some probation officers actively encourage the formation of probation/parolees' organizations and ex-offenders' association, for the purposes of mutual assistance in their rehabilitation efforts and advocacy in improving probation programmes and services;

- probationers are encouraged to organize co-operatives or to join an existing co-operative in their neighbourhood, for the purpose of securing loans, gaining access to markets

> for their products and assuring a steady supply of raw materials or clients for their business or services;
>
> • probation officers link up with religious organizations, schools and civic groups to provide their clients with opportunities to attend seminars on value formation and spiritual renewal, personality development and family relations, and to receive literacy training and non-formal education.
>
> (Written by Francisco C. Ruivivar, Administrator, Parole and Probation Administration, Department of Justice, the Philippines)

ROLE CONFLICT

The final section of this chapter considers the issue of role conflict between the control and care functions of probation. Managing the inherent tension between the control and care components of supervising offenders in the community has always been difficult. The original concept of probation combined the conditional suspension of punishment with the provision of help and support. The most obvious form of tension arises when the offender ignores the conditions on which punishment was suspended. At a philosophical level there is no difficulty in reconciling care and control in these circumstances, but in terms of sustaining a productive personal relationship with the offender, there obviously can be.

Some country experts referred to the tensions which arise between pursuing the interests of the offender and those of the broader community, especially where, as in Japan, probation officers have an explicit crime preventive role, as well as a rehabilitative one. Where probation systems have developed from the classic model towards correctionalism, there would seem to be scope for additional forms of role conflict. The more that probation supervision is intended to serve multiple functions – rehabilitation, reparation, retribution – the more scope there is for confusion and tension. For example, in England and Wales greater emphasis has been placed – at least on the part of central government – on the deprivation of liberty involved in serving probation orders. Whilst this helps locate probation more coherently with a deserts-based sentencing framework, attempts to ensure that supervision does genuinely serve a secondary, retributive function in curtailing the offender's freedom of action could create as many problems as they solve.

Though the experts in the majority of the countries recognized the potential for role conflict, they reported remarkably few problems in, for example, Australia, Hungary, the Philippines, Papua New Guinea or Scotland. The notable exception was in England and Wales. Here there was a perceived conflict, with many rank-and-file probation officers thinking that the policies of the Home Office and senior probation management were displacing traditional social work functions with more controlling and punitive supervision. The lack of consensus about the right balance to be struck seemed to be significantly limiting the capabilities of the Probation Service. Why this should be so is unclear. What is clear is that other developed countries, such as Australia, have managed to shift their probation systems in the correctionalist direction without creating the same turbulences. Possible explanations of the difficulties in England and Wales include:

• that the system is heavily professionalized, with a working ethos firmly grounded in social work practice;
• that the very size and age of the service engenders a degree of conservatism;
• that the political distance between the main probation union and the government of the day would jeopardize any but the blandest of the latter's initiatives; and
• that the reluctance of the workforce to move in the correctionalist direction has prompted a vicious spiral of managerialist interventions which fuel further reluctance.

The precise mix of ingredients is less important for our purposes than the question whether role conflict is necessarily exacerbated in systems which shift their focus from treatment to correctionalism. The answer, at least on the basis of our sample, is that it is not.

Chapter 8

Volunteer probation personnel

Koichi Hamai and Renaud Villé

This chapter is concerned with the use of volunteers within the probation systems covered by the study. In some countries volunteers play an important role in the probation service, not only in relieving the pressure of work on probation officers but also in stimulating community participation in criminal justice and facilitating the reintegration of offenders in the community.

Table 8.1 summarizes the type of use made within the twelve systems. Only three make no use of volunteers – New South Wales, Hungary and Israel. Of the nine that do, seven have statutory provision for the use of volunteers. Table 8.2 summarizes the benefits accruing to volunteers in the different systems. Table 8.3 shows the criteria for eligibility as a volunteer. The remainder of the chapter considers the use of volunteers by each of the nine systems in turn.

AUSTRALIA (SOUTH AUSTRALIA)

The Department has had an active volunteer programme since the mid-1970s. Volunteers are used in a wide range of prison and community corrections programmes and activities, and service as a volunteer has often been a trigger to social work training and subsequent employment as probation officer or correctional officer.

Volunteers are involved in work with individual clients, group-work, programme work and providing support to offenders and their families in prison and the community in areas such as literacy, social skills, transport, general support for clients and their families, art and craft courses, driver training, basic mechanics, sewing, cooking, Aboriginal culture craft and recreational activities.

Table 8.1 Types of use of volunteers

	Status		Type of use			
	Y/N	Legislation	Formal policy	Ad hoc	Mix	Systematic
New South Wales	No					
South Australia	Yes	X		X		X
Western Australia	Yes	X				
Canada	Yes		X		X	X
Hungary	No	X		X		
Israel	No					
Japan	Yes	X				X
Papua New Guinea	Yes	X		X		
The Philippines	Yes	X				X
Sweden	Yes	X		X		
England and Wales	Yes				X	
Scotland	Yes		X			

Notes: 'No' means that no volunteer probation personnel are utilized. A cross (X) indicates what probation system in each country is classified in terms of the status and the type of use of volunteers.

Table 8.2 Compensation for volunteers

| | Compensation | | | | | Step |
	Remuneration	Reimbursement	Status	Certificate	Seminar	
South Australia		X	X	X	X	No
Western Australia		X				No
Canada						
Japan		X	X	X	X	No
Papua New Guinea		X	X			No
The Philippines		X	X	X	X	No
Sweden	X	X				No
England and Wales						Yes
Scotland		X				Yes

Notes: (1) The following abbreviations are used in the table: Remuneration (financial compensation for the activities of volunteers excluding reimbursement for expenses incurred during their duties); Reimbursement (reimbursement for expenses incurred during the duties of volunteers such as postage, telephone and travel); Status (officially recognized professional status with some identification cards); Certificate (official recognition and appreciation awarded by authorities); Seminar (opportunity to participate in training course, seminar and/or workshop); Step (step towards employment as a probation officer as the result of their services as a volunteer). (2) Although a remuneration is offered in Sweden, this is very limited, and cannot be regarded as a wage.

Table 8.3 Requirements for volunteers

	Maximum age	Minimum age	Exam	No criminal record
South Australia	X			
Western Australia				X
Canada		X		
Japan		X		X
Papua New Guinea	X	X		X
The Philippines		X	X	X
Sweden				
England and Wales				
Scotland				

Volunteers are not used in a formed capacity, for example as honorary probation officers, though there is statutory provision for the use of volunteers. Section 8 of the Correctional Services Act 1982 (the legislation governing the administration of the prisons, home detention, parole and community service programmes) states that: 'The Minister must promote the use of volunteers in the administration of this Act to such extent as the Minister may authorise.' There are just under sixty volunteers at present.

Volunteers are selected on the basis of the experience and skills that they bring into the Department. To be selected, volunteers need to be reliable, realistic and at the same time have empathy for clients and to be good communicators. They are trained by the staff of the Volunteer Unit. The (compulsory) training course draws in staff members from the Department with special areas of expertise. About forty volunteers are trained a year.

Volunteers are only paid out-of-pocket expenses. This is usually payment for use of private motor car mileage and fares for public transport. They are provided with accreditation and an identification card which provides them with access to all Departmental facilities. Certificates of recognition are presented for five, ten and fifteen years' continuous service. Training is provided for probation officers to ensure appropriate use and support of volunteers. There are bi-monthly meetings with staff and volunteers, who also attend staff meetings at Community Correctional Centres.

A number of volunteers have gone on to obtain professional qualifications and as result have been offered a position as probation officer. However, service as a volunteer is not a necessary requirement for such an appointment.

AUSTRALIA (WESTERN AUSTRALIA)

The function of volunteers is similar to community corrections officers, but they are supervised closely by CCOs. They have all the statutory powers of government-employed CCOs and are called honorary community corrections officers. Most honorary community corrections officers are attached to country areas rather than metropolitan offices. Careful selection ensures good working relationships. It is left up to the individual Community Correction Centre manager to recruit as needed. No information on the number of honorary probation officers is available.

Under the community corrections legislation (Offenders Community Correction Act 1963) the chief executive officer may appoint any person, not being a member of the police force, to be an honorary community corrections officer and at any time may remove any person so appointed. Though mature people are preferred, there is no formal minimum or maximum age. Volunteers have to be respected community members, with skills which the service can make use of. There are no formal training courses. Managers of individual Community Correction Centres may arrange informal training, which is encouraged but not compulsory.

Volunteers are reimbursed for expenses like travel, phone calls and postage. There are no other entitlements. Serving as a volunteer is not a step towards employment as a probation officer. Some sessional supervisors (i.e. paid casual part-time employees, mostly responsible for work order supervision) have filled temporary vacancies, but all permanent positions which become vacant must be advertised for competitive selection.

CANADA

All provinces use volunteers in the probation service except Quebec and Yukon. Newfoundland has an Assistant Probation Officer Programme where contractual services are sought in geographically remote communities. Nova Scotia has about 150 registered volunteers and 27 paraprofessionals. The paraprofessionals are called assistant probation officers and are not considered to be volunteers. They supervise a small token caseload (approximately twenty) and perform other duties such as pre-sentence report preparation, court attendance, case supervision and alternative measure hearings, on a contractual fee for service basis.

Probation volunteers in Canada perform the following tasks:

- supervision (Prince Edward Island, Nova Scotia, New Brunswick, Ontario, Manitoba, Saskatchewan, Alberta, North-West Territories);
- PSRs (Prince Edward Island, Ontario, Manitoba);
- programme assistance (Prince Edward Island, Nova Scotia, New Brunswick, Ontario, Manitoba, Saskatchewan, Alberta, British Columbia);
- counselling (Prince Edward Island, Nova Scotia, Ontario, Saskatchewan, Alberta, North-West Territories);
- administrative support (Nova Scotia, Ontario, Manitoba, Alberta);
- court (Prince Edward Island, Nova Scotia, Ontario, Saskatchewan, Alberta);
- recreation programmes (Prince Edward Island, Manitoba).

The principal concern in selecting volunteers is that they should be responsible and effective people who are going to be of assistance to the probation service. There is no hard and fast prohibition of persons with criminal records being volunteers, but there is concern that the possibility of additional offending is minimized. There is particular concern about sexual offenders. Nova Scotia indicates that volunteers are required to take orientation training from supervising probation officers; this is compulsory for new volunteers. The training covers background information regarding the purpose and structure of corrections, the department, interviewing skills and orientation to offenders.

HUNGARY

Volunteers were used until 1992 in the work of both juvenile and adult probation officers. The modification of the Penal Code abolished this, and the work of volunteers has to be put on a new basis in the adult probation system. This modification abolished the institution of reformatory work, a kind of punishment executed at the offenders' place of employment. Its task was to help the offender to adapt to the society with the help of his/her fellow-workers, and in addition during the punishment the convict earned less, so it was considered to be a kind of fine. Some of these fellow-workers really wanted to help the offenders and become volunteers for this purpose. Then this kind of volunteer worker disappeared. The use of volunteers is provided for in the legislation, but because of the dramatically economic changes in the country very few people apply to be volunteers.

JAPAN

Volunteer probation officers play a very significant part within the Japanese probation and parole system; there are almost 50,000 of them. The roles of volunteer probation officers are to help the rehabilitation of offenders within the community and to encourage public support for and involvement in, crime prevention. The Offender Rehabilitation Law (1949) prescribes the use of volunteer probation officers who act as government agents in the rehabilitation service. The Volunteer Probation Officer Law (1950) describes the qualification, selection, duties and other relevant aspects of the volunteer probation officers.

Volunteers' key function in dealing with offenders is supervising and helping probationers and parolees, who are assigned to them on an individual basis. But they also have various other duties, which include: visits to inmates' homes to keep the family informed and to prepare reports for the probation office as a part of pre-release preparation; locating probationers or parolees who have moved in from another area and taking over supervisory casework with them; preliminary investigation of candidates for pardons; and assistance to the offender's family.

On the crime prevention side, volunteers carry out a variety of activities relating to community organization, including collaboration with public and private organizations to explore and mobilize social resources in the community; explaining the philosophy of rehabilitation to individual neighbours or the public as a whole; and tackling – in co-operation with community residents – criminogenic environmental conditions.

The recruitment of suitable candidates is not an easy task. The director of the probation office is responsible for preparing a list of candidates on the basis of information he/she has gathered from various sources in the community. The list largely reflects the views of representatives of the VPO Associations. Further screening is made of the list of applicants by an advisory committee which the law prescribes should consist of not more than fifteen members, consisting of representatives of justice, prosecution, the bar, institutional correction, probation and parole and other public commissions as well as 'learned citizens'. The candidates who pass such screening are then appointed as VPOs by the Minister of Justice.

The qualities required of a volunteer probation officer are stated in the Volunteer Probation Officer Law as: confidence and recognition in the community with respect to his/her personality and conduct; enthusiasm and time for such work; financial stability; and good health. Each probation office to which volunteer probation officers are appointed is expected to orga- nize and conduct training which is compulsory. There are three initial training courses for volunteers, one for newly appointed volunteer probation officers, one for all second year volunteers and a further course for those with three or four years' experi- ence. In addition, there are some refresher courses for those with several years' experience. Each year, about 2,500 people are newly appointed as volunteer probation officers, which is about five per cent of the total. The duration of the training course varies from one- to three-day sessions. Initial training covers criminology and criminal justice policy; the rehabilitation and aftercare system; supervision of probationers and parolees; preparation of offenders for release; crime prevention activities. Additional training is available in specific professional skills. To supplement this the Japan Rehabilitation Aid Association publishes a monthly periodical entitled *Rehabilitation*, which is intended to help volunteers acquire the knowledge and skills they need.

EXPERIENCE OF A VOLUNTEER PROBATION OFFICER IN JAPAN

What follows is an account of one probationer in Japan related by a volunteer probation officer. It illustrates the role of the volunteer probation officer in Japan, since the story shows how volunteer probation officers supervise offenders, how they help offenders (mediating between the offender and the local commu- nity) and how they co-operate with probation officers.

Tadashi is 26 years old. Although he is not an active person, he has a short temper and has shown his impatience and carelessness on many occasions. He dropped out of school when he was 17 years of age and changed his employment many times during a brief period of time. He violated traffic laws several times and also caused traffic accidents on two occasions which resulted in the withdrawal of his driving licence. Because of the loss of his driver's licence he lost his job and gradually became involved with the Yakuza (a Japanese organized crime ring).

After several months he was a fully-fledged member of the Yakuza and involved in their illegal activities: he had also had his chest tattooed. He was then arrested by the police with the charge of illegal possession and the selling of drugs and received a probation order from the court. As a volunteer probation officer, I was assigned the task of supervising him by my probation officer, who is in charge of the supervision of all the probationers in my area.

During the legal process, Tadashi realized the meaning of what he had done and decided to leave the Yakuza and to become a law-abiding member of the community. However, since it is very difficult to leave the Yakuza once you have become a member, he was always afraid of being found and taken back to the Yakuza and expressed this fear to me during a visit to my house for a supervisory session.

I encouraged him to be strong willed, but I also realized that it was not easy and I had to do something to help him. I decided to consult my supervising probation officer and asked his assistance with this problem. The probation officer contacted the police and found that the boss of the Yakuza group which Tadashi had joined had also been arrested and was detained in prison. The probation officer, in collaboration with the staff of the prison, negotiated with the boss about giving Tadashi permission to leave the organization, and then finally received the boss's written approval.

When I informed Tadashi and his family of the boss's decision, the gratitude and pleasure shown by both Tadashi and his family was impossible to express. Tadashi was greatly encouraged by this approval and began to have a positive attitude towards his future. He obtained another driver's licence within three months and worked very hard as a construction worker. I noted that every time he visited my home he had become both physically and psychologically tougher with a positive outlook on life.

Several months later, however, he was rather upset when he was asked by his little niece to show her the tattoo he had on his chest, since he still had the tattoo which was a kind of symbol of the Yakuza. The tattoo made him feel ashamed since it reminded him of his past. He very much regretted the fact that he had tattooed his skin, and cried and said to me that he would do anything to remove the tattoo. In view of this, I asked several doctors whom I know and was introduced to a surgeon, a Dr Tanaka, who is very experienced. I made an appointment with Dr Tanaka and went to see him with Tadashi. The doctor understood the situation and said he would like to co-operate with us, but since the operation would be very expensive, Tadashi must first of all speak to his parents with regard to paying for the operation. Tadashi consulted them saying that he would stop smoking and gambling and would return the money to them later. They finally agreed to pay for the surgery. Tadashi entered hospital and had to have three operations to remove the tattoo since it was very big. He stayed in the hospital for three months.

After his release from the hospital, he started looking for employment and although he searched hard and enthusiastically for a job, it was not so easy to find a position. Therefore, in order to help him I also consulted a friend who owns a small company. My friend told me that the position in his company required a lot of physical effort and may be too hard for a person who had just been released from hospital. However, he suggested that Tadashi obtain a licence to enable him to drive a lorry or large vehicle and introduced him to a shipping company.

After one month, he got this driver's licence and started working as a long-distance truck driver and every time he came to my house, he told me of the places he had visited.

At the same time, I continued discussing drug problems with Tadashi according to the Treatment Guidelines for Drug-related Offenders issued by the Probation Department.

Since Tadashi continued to work hard and did not violate any probation conditions over a long period of time, I proposed to my probation officer that Tadashi receive a temporary discharge probation order. After an interview with my probation officer, Tadashi was temporally discharged from his probation order.Three years later, Tadashi is still working at the same company.

Source: Translation of the case study written by Mrs Kikuko Fukuoka and published in the *Japanese Journal of Rehabilitation*, August 1993.

Volunteer probation officers are reimbursed for all or part of expenses incurred in discharging their duty. In practice, they are reimbursed a certain amount irrespective of actual expenditure; as of 1993, a maximum of 4,630 yen per month (about US$45) for supervising a probationer or parolee and 1,200 yen for a report on the home environment to which the inmate will return from prison. There are no other entitlements.

It can be seen, therefore, that the material benefits from serving as a VPO hardly serve as an incentive. As in any other field of voluntary work, what motivates a VPO is the sense of mission, and the gratification he/she derives from seeing a good response to the help he/she provides. Social prestige attached to being a volunteer may be an additional incentive to some extent, especially since public recognition of individual VPOs' achievements is regularly given in the form of certificates and honours.

PAPUA NEW GUINEA

Under the Probation Act VPOs assist and befriend a probationer. When required they prepare and submit written reports in respect of a probationer. Volunteers who do not read or write give verbal reports to the probation officer who then writes up the report. Generally the VPO assists the probation officer in the performance of his/her duties. The task of taking formal action against offenders who have breached their conditions of probation is done by a probation officer and not a VPO.

There are just under 300 active VPOs. They come from the community the offender lives in. From talking and listening to the offender's family, close relatives and other influential community members the VPO becomes a catalyst in getting the community to support the probationer in ways which will change and improve his/her behaviour, and thus prevent reoffending.

Volunteers should be of mature age, good character and a respected member of the community. The shape of VPO training is specified by Head Office's training section; provincial probation and parole officers actually plan and conduct the workshops or courses. After completion of training VPOs are awarded certificates of achievement. Although this training is not compulsory, all VPOs are encouraged to undertake it. Approximately 50 per cent of VPOs do some form of training each year. The normal maximum training course period is three days. There is initial training for volunteers. It covers VPO duties and responsibilities under the legislation, the Probation Service organization and its policies, the criminal justice system and where the probation system fits within it. There is training in specific skills for volunteers covering counselling and interviewing skills.

Working relationships between volunteers and officers are very good. There is an initial tendency for volunteers to take too simplistic a view of probation work, but this is overcome as they learn the role of the Probation Service within the criminal justice system.

Volunteers are reimbursed for expenses incurred while performing their duties. After completion of a VPO induction course the chief probation officer gives them a certificate of achievement. This certificate is useful when it becomes necessary for him/her to visit a police lock-up to check for a probationer. Serving as a volunteer is not a step towards employment as a probation officer.

THE PHILIPPINES

The statutory duty of probation aides (volunteers) is to assist provincial or city probation officers in the supervision of probationers and parolees. Their specific duties vary from one regional office to another but generally include the following:

- helping paid staff supervise clients, especially in inaccessible country areas;
- guidance and counselling;
- helping offenders get employment;
- advocacy and information dissemination about the probation programme;
- organizing/supervising religious activities, athletics competitions, cultural activities.

The use of volunteers is provided for in the law and probation rules. Generally, volunteers are assigned clients to supervise on a one-to-one basis, but not exceeding five clients at any one time. They work under the close supervision of regular staff. In 1992 680 volunteers were recruited, 330 were trained, 125 were appointed; a total of 758 were in active service as of 31 December 1992.

The law provides that the probation administrator may appoint citizens of good repute and probity to act as probation aides to assist the probation and parole officers in the supervision of probationers and parolees. The power to appoint probation aides (volunteers) is now delegated to the regional directors, including the power to set the qualifications of said volunteers within the statutory limits and to determine the period they can hold office. Generally, the minimum age required is 21 years, and the volunteer should have no criminal record. Some regions give special examinations to applicants. A study of volunteers showed that 57 per cent were males, 50 per cent were college graduates and 29 per cent college undergraduates; 68 per cent were married; 68 per cent were employed and 10.4 per cent were students; 18 per cent were below 26 years old, 61 per cent belonged to the age group 26-49 years old; and 21 per cent were 50 years old or above. There are no formal training courses for volunteers, though chief probation and parole officers of each field office give orientation lectures and on-the-job training to volunteers on a needs basis.

The volunteer programme is perceived with some ambivalence by probation officers. Although the majority accept the validity of the programme and the benefits of employing volunteers, more than 50 per cent of all probation offices do not employ volunteers. Some are wary about assigning control functions to volunteers and would rather limit their work to the assistance/care functions. However, in those offices which employ volunteers, probation officers appreciate their usefulness in supervising probationers and parolees, especially in those offices that are under-manned, or those in inaccessible areas with poor public transport, such as islands and mountainous regions.

Although volunteers do not receive any regular compensation for their services, they may be given a reasonable travel allowance. The amount is determined by the regional director within the limits set by accounting rules and regulations. The entitlement and incentives to facilitate the work or motivate the volunteers vary from one regional office to another, but generally include formal appointment as a volunteer probation aide and an accompanying identification card. Volunteers are generally treated as members of the probation staff, and invited to participate in group activities and assist in public information seminars on probation. Recognition of the services of volunteers is also effected through certificates or plaques of appreciation and recognition awarded by the chief probation and parole officer, by the regional director, or by the administrator depending on the value of the contribution made to the Parole and Probation Administration. Such awards are usually given on special occasions such as anniversaries or annual meetings.

Service as a volunteer is generally not a step towards employment as a probation officer. The qualification standards for employment as probation officers are much higher than those for probation volunteers. However, this does not preclude qualified volunteers from applying for employment as probation officer. There are some probation officers who were former volunteers.

SWEDEN

The staff resources of the probation service include nonprofessional lay supervisors, who are given guidance and support by probation officers. Probation officers use lay supervisors rather than take on supervision themselves in 45 per cent of cases. In these cases, probation officers must maintain some contact with the offender. The probation officer must meet the client and the lay supervisor within a month of the passing of the sentence for a planning interview.

Lay supervisors are appointed by the court or by the chief probation officer. There are roughly 4,500 active at any one time. Their contact with clients is not directly regulated by statute with regard to frequency or content. The law provides in general terms that the client shall keep the supervisor informed about his/her circumstances of employment and accommodation, present him- or herself when called for and follow instructions. Supervisors help clients develop their everyday social skills and also serve as a link to the community. No special qualifications, profession or social position are necessary to become a lay supervisor. The client has a right to suggest a certain person as his/her supervisor. If this suggestion is reasonable, it is usually granted. The probation officer and the lay supervisor divide up the work with clients in accordance with the nature of the case. The probation officer has a general responsibility for supervising the activities of the volunteer and providing advice and support. Usually the probation officer gets more involved in the control function and in liaising with other authorities while the lay supervisor works more as a befriender and role-model. The division of labour is discussed and settled at the outset of the supervision period, but is often revised.

It is thought desirable that lay supervisors should meet the clients they are supervising once or twice a week at least at the start of supervision, though contact rates vary considerably. The meeting place will very often be the home of either the client or the lay supervisor but it may also be a public place.

Volunteers should be interested in people and in social issues, and have rounded personalities. The Probation Service can arrange training, though this is not compulsory. It typically comprises eight to ten sessions lasting two to three hours. The Probation Service offers volunteers additional training in the form of courses, lectures and discussions on such matters as social issues, legislation, supervision methods and drug abuse problems. Again, this training is not compulsory.

Lay supervisors receive 200 kroner per month (roughly US$ 26), half of this being for expenses incurred, half as fee. In addition they may claim reimbursement for long journeys, loss of earnings and other special costs subject to the probation officer's approval, e.g. where specially intensive activity by the supervisor is needed for a given period and for a special purpose such as help with studies, daily home visits or introduction to a caring institution. There is no other entitlement, and serving as a volunteer is not a step towards employment as a probation officer.

Though lay supervisors can provide an effective complement to probation officers, opinion is fairly equally divided amongst officers themselves as to their value. Some think that supervisors do a very good job, whilst others see them as a source of additional work and trouble.

UNITED KINGDOM (ENGLAND AND WALES)

Until the late 1960s volunteer involvement was largely limited to prison visiting and aftercare support, but over the last two decades volunteers have become much more widely used. Indeed, some experience of voluntary work within the probation service is almost a prerequisite for being accepted on probation training courses, and the majority of probation students supported by the Home Office will have worked as volunteers.

Volunteers are involved in work with individual clients, group-work, providing transport, and support for families when a member is in custody. Research carried out in the mid-1980s suggested a degree of ambivalence towards volunteers on the part of probation officers and underutilization of their potential.

There are no nationally set requirements, though volunteers would invariably be interviewed before being accepted. The responsibility for training rests with local probation areas. Provision varies widely. The training is compulsory in the sense that normally volunteers would be approved by an area only after they had received some induction training. The duration of the training course varies. There is initial training for volunteers, but no training in specific skills. There is no statutory provision for the use of volunteers, nor are there any relevant national policy statements or standards. No information is held centrally about numbers of volunteers. Volunteers receive no financial compensation.

UNITED KINGDOM (SCOTLAND)

The use of volunteers is a matter of policy, not of law. Volunteers undertake a wide variety of tasks concerned with the rehabilitation of offenders, mostly as members of independent sector organizations, rather than local authorities. These tasks include:

- befriending individual offenders and/or their families;
- assisting individual offenders with welfare tasks;
- providing help to individual offenders or groups of offenders with literacy or other educational needs;
- providing transport for families visiting prisoners;
- assisting with the running of prison visitors centres, libraries in prisons, etc;
- acting as members of the management committees of voluntary bodies set up to assist offenders;
- acting as mediators in mediation and reparation schemes;
- providing counselling in alcohol and drugs;
- providing support for victims of crime.

Volunteers do not have formal responsibility for supervising offenders on behalf of the court. They work usually in support of local authority efforts through their participation in independent sector agencies. The National Standards encourage local authorities to make the most effective use of existing voluntary sector agencies and to stimulate new initiatives from these agencies where appropriate.

There are no nationally set requirements for volunteers in the social service field. Requirements are set by the agencies who use them. Nor is there a national strategy or programme for the training of volunteers working in social services, including criminal justice social services. This is a matter for each agency, and each does it differently. Basic training is compulsory in most agencies using volunteers extensively in the criminal justice system, but further training is not. The duration of training courses is variable – from a few hours to twelve days. Those agencies which provide systematic training are likely to cover at least some of the following: interviewing skills; counselling skills; listening skills; giving and receiving information; communication skills; sharing information; coping with relapse; and handling aggression.

Volunteers are normally reimbursed for travel and other incidental costs linked to their work. Serving as a volunteer is a step towards employment as a probation officer for the following reasons:

• some volunteers develop an interest in this area of work and then decide to seek a qualification;
• others may deliberately take up voluntary work with a view to enhancing their chances of obtaining a place on a qualifying course in social work;
• volunteers can take certain elements of the SVQ (Scottish Vocational Qualification) by way of preparation for entry into qualifying training.

Chapter 9

Reflections on comparative probation

Robert Harris

The study of comparative law does not aim at the discovery of the nearest equivalent, in one system, of a particular detail of a legal rule or provision in another. Rather do such studies try to demonstrate the limited number of possibilities available for the solution of similar social problems. ... The more references to concrete particulars are omitted and the wider the range of the underlying conception, the more comparability and unity among different national systems will be achieved.

(United Nations 1959: 1–2)

The study reported in Part II contains information about probation systems in Australia, Canada, England and Wales, Hungary, Israel, Japan, Papua New Guinea, the Philippines, Scotland and Sweden. This chapter selects for discussion key points from the data provided and offers preliminary comparative observations.

We have already sounded a note of caution about the quality of some of our data and its robustness as a basis for comparative study. In doing so we were acknowledging the limitations under which the study was conducted, which involved necessarily depending on single case studies by local experts whose access to comparative data was limited and who were reliant on statistics which were sometimes incomplete or of limited reliability. This caveat is reiterated here, though our concerns about data quality do not vitiate the value of the study as a whole: its general thrust is correct though verification of some details has proved impossible and we have encountered minor inconsistencies.

We should also mention the technical problem of dealing with Australia and Canada, where probation policy and administration are devolved to states or provinces, with differences existing among them. In this chapter references to Australia and Canada are generalizations, and readers who wish for greater precision should refer back to earlier chapters. On the few occasions where significant interstate differences exist they are noted, but federal law is on the whole sufficiently strong to create reasonable cohesion among state or provincial legislation, and most differences are of detail not principle.

In this chapter no attempt is made to summarize the preceding chapters in Part II, but we extract and comment on key points in each, drawing also on data not mentioned previously, but deriving from discussion with national experts or supporting documentation.[1]

SOME CHARACTERISTICS OF PROBATION IN THE CASE STUDY COUNTRIES

The probation order

The *age of criminal responsibility* (and hence at which the probation service may become involved with juveniles) varies in our countries between 9 and 14. There is no official involvement with juveniles in Sweden, Scotland and parts of Australia – as in Hungary and the Philippines, any such involvement is distinct from work with adults; and in many countries probation's role with juveniles is subsidiary to that of other agencies, ranging from the well-organized statutory or voluntary welfare services of Western Europe to the semi-official but community-based youth groups found in Eastern Europe and Japan. In all countries, however, probation officers deal with adults, in most cases from the age of 18.

Throughout the world probation is predominantly for *middle-range offenders*. Though there may be slight differences of emphasis the category normally embraces property offences where aggravation was not involved, non-grievous acts of violence, criminal damage of a more than trivial kind, car theft and many non-penetrative sexual offences. In all countries except Sweden our experts claim probation is used also for minor offences; Sweden is excluded because conditional

sentences, of which probation is one, can be used only for imprisonable offences; though the same restriction applies in Hungary,
there the scale of imprisonable offences itself embraces more
minor crimes.

Most countries permit probation to be used for serious offences,
normally where extenuating circumstances exist. A trend for
probation to be used alongside other controlling measures as an
alternative to custody is increasingly discernible. Electronic monitoring is in widespread use in Canada, Australia and the United
States, and is under active consideration in Sweden and England
and Wales; in Australia the very name probation has largely given
way to community corrections; in Canada a similar possibility was
for a while under active consideration.

Apart from Sweden, where probation is of standard length,
probation is of variable duration. Where specified, minimum
periods are for six months or a year with maxima normally three
years, the exceptions being Japan and some Australian states
(which permit five-year orders), and PNG and the Philippines,
where six-year orders are possible. In the cases of Hungary, Japan
and the Philippines, however, the length of probation relates to
the length of the prison sentence for which it is a substitute. This
renders PNG unique in the sample in permitting a six-year probation sentence in its own right, a policy which is the more surprising
since probation for serious offences is rare, and there appears no
concept of probation unyoked from supervision. Elsewhere, seemingly influenced by studies which suggest a declining rate of return
for long-term professional contact (such studies began with Reid
and Shyne 1970; for a recent review of the literature on short-
term intervention with alcohol misusers in particular see Bien *et
al.* 1993) there is a trend for intervention to be shorter, but more
focused and purposive.

Data which invite *comparison of probation and custody rates*
do not present a clear picture. In the majority of case study
countries the trends are for probation numbers to increase steadily
rather than spectacularly. Of countries where the rise has been
steep, PNG's exponential increases are perhaps to be expected:
the service began only in 1985 and absolute numbers remain small.
Of more significance is Canada where, after plateauing around
66,000–73,000 between 1986 and 1989 probation numbers rose to
83,000 in 1991 and 93,000 in 1992. Though one must be cautious
in extrapolating, the increases have coincided with economic

recession, increasing political sensitivity to the costs of prison places and a fall in the prison population. Though slight in 1991 this fall was considerable in 1992, a year which saw the numbers of probation orders move from 32,000 *less* than the numbers of prison sentences in 1991 to 18,000 *more*.

Other countries (Israel, Scotland) have seen upward trends in both prison and probation sentences over time; only Japan has witnessed a significant decline in both: between 1980 and 1991 the number of probation orders fell by 43 per cent while prison sentences fell by 30 per cent. Again one must be cautious in interpreting these figures, though it is clear that for a country with a low crime rate and innumerable informal mechanisms of crime control (Moriyama 1989) the rate of imprisonment has been slightly higher than is sometimes believed: even in 1991 for example, the ratio of prison:probation sentences was over 4:1, a figure exceeded in our study only by Israel. On the face of it this sits uneasily with the view of Japan as a country where attitudes towards offenders are rendered non-punitive by social processes such as reintegrative shaming (Braithwaite 1989: 61–5).

All case study countries permit sentencers latitude in making *additional requirements* to probation orders (or their equivalent). This illustrates the limited purchase today of the argument discussed in Chapter 2 that imposing requirements on offenders beyond those enshrined in law was contrary to civil liberty. It demonstrates also the diminution of opposition, popular as well as intellectual, to discipline and surveillance at the very time when such surveillance is more technologically feasible (Foucault 1977; Cohen 1985; Harris and Webb 1987: Chapter 7).

Organization and structure

With the exception of Hungary, where juvenile probation officers are employed by local communities themselves and adult officers by courts, *responsibility for probation* falls between national and local (or state/provincial) government. It is clear, however, that these responses in some cases simplify a more complex situation. For example:

- in England and Wales probation officers have conditions of employment similar but not identical to those of *local* government employees, are 80 per cent funded by *central* government, but are employees of neither, being employed by committees/boards comprising local councillors, magistrates, experts and members of the community;

- in PNG, though core funding is from central government and accountability is to the Attorney-General's Department of the Ministry for Justice, the service is dependent on subventions from community and provincial governments, and has also received support from sources as diverse as churches, businesses and the Canadian High Commission.

In the light of the fact that in more than one country probation services have been described as being 'servants to two masters', we explored the *relationship of probation to the courts*. Only in Hungary do courts actually fund the officers, so combining accountability with resourcing. More frequently, and consistent with their normal constitutional role as instruments not originators of criminal policy, courts are controllers not employers, able to demand service but not determine policy. The Australian system is fairly typical: probation officers are 'not directly employed by the courts but could be described as "officers of the court"' (New South Wales) and 'prepare reports for the Courts and supervise offenders on Court imposed orders' (South Australia).

We sought to ascertain the *balance between professionalism and bureaucracy* in different probation systems. The Israeli service is the most traditionally professional in that its officers 'enjoy organizational and professional autonomy ... serve the courts and law enforcement agencies in the capacity of professional advisor, and are so recognized'.[2] Elsewhere, however, probation's increasingly central role has combined with the demise of confidence in the clinical treatment of offenders to reduce respectively its organizational and professional autonomy, emphasizing instead the firmness of its position within local justice delivery systems.

The majority of probation services claim to have a *union or professional association* available to staff, though such organizations vary:

- national associations for probation staff exist in England and Wales, Hungary, the Philippines and Sweden;
- similar provincial or state associations, which are in some cases defined subsets of public sector unions or associations, are found

in New South Wales, South Australia, Ontario, Nova Scotia and
New Brunswick;
- social work organizations which probation staff are eligible to
  join exist in Israel and Scotland;
- civil service or similar associations which probation officers
  may join by dint of employment status not professional affiliation are reported as existing in Western Australia and Japan,
  though given their employment status this option seems likely
  to be more generally available to probation officers round the
  world.

Though New South Wales, Ontario, Quebec, the Philippines
and Scotland claim to have a code of ethics, monitoring and
enforcement appear limited: nowhere could we uncover evidence
of disciplinary procedures relating to professional misconduct as
distinct from breaches of the terms and conditions of employment. Indeed it is not clear how meaningful any such distinction
could be.

The *minimum educational level* required for probation officers
varies, though in practice except in PNG over half of all
officers are graduates. Excluding Australia, where differences
are wide, five countries require a first degree (though the best
qualified probation service we have encountered is in Prince
Edward Island, where a masters degree is necessary); most
(the exceptions being Hungary and PNG) require a professional
qualification or an examination. In PNG the emphasis is on
personal qualities and motivation; in Hungary economic circumstances gravitate against such requirements, even volunteers being
hard to find:

> It is very difficult to find anyone who wants or is able to help.
> Unemployment is very high, lots of people have no job, no
> home, no existence: that is why people, and society in general
> do not want to help these deviant persons.

> Probation officers have no budget, so they cannot give material
> aid to offenders to help them live or eat.

Only Hungary lacks *compulsory initial training*, though
such training is variably located. A direct professional association
with social work is becoming rare. Only in South Australia, Israel,
England and Wales and Scotland is it normally located in
university schools of social work, though in Sweden many officers

transfer from such schools. Elsewhere initial training is in-house and of varying lengths (two to four weeks in Canada, one month in the Philippines, six weeks in PNG, three months in New South Wales and nine months in Japan).

Though course content varies from a cursory introduction in Canada to a thorough programme in Japan, the main focus is on setting the work of the probation officer into its organizational and judicial context, and providing practical information on 'how to do the job'. In Japan training contains elements of criminology, behavioural science and counselling; in PNG it covers interviewing and counselling, and supervising VPOs.

Most countries provide post-experience training, though it is of varying length and content, and differentially available: in South Australia up to 70 per cent of staff receive such training in any one year, whereas in Japan the figure is 5 per cent (70 officers out of a workforce of 1,440). Training is sometimes compulsory sometimes not, content varies widely, as does the importance attached to it. In England and Wales, though responsibility for such training lies with local services, increasing concern about training has caused the Home Office to institute a Probation Training Unit with responsibility for co-ordinating and monitoring training policies as a whole; the Philippine expert specifically related attendance at such events to career advancement:

> Training in specific skills received is considered important for career advancement as it upgrades the skills of the employee, increases efficiency and effectiveness in his/her work, increases his/her contribution to the productivity of the organization, and hence, improves the prospects for promotion.

To try to comprehend the status of probation officers from another angle we enquired about *salary levels in relation to other professions* which constitute a possible reference group: teachers, nurses and police, and about salaries *vis-à-vis* the average national male industrial wage. In all countries probation officers were paid more than nurses and the average wage; in PNG, the Philippines and parts of Australia probation officers were the highest paid of these professions; in every other country probation officers earned less than the police; in Israel, Japan and Sweden they also earned less than state school teachers.

Functions

We were interested in the *stages in the criminal justice process in which the probation service was involved*. In all countries other than Japan and the Philippines involvement begins prior to trial or sentence in a reporting function or (particularly in Australia, Israel and Great Britain) for bail assessment or supervision. In Japan probation referrals are made only after sentence, and in the Philippines, probation being imposed only on application and in lieu of the execution of a prison sentence, the same applies – though the post-sentence report is likely to be influential in determining whether probation is to be offered.

All services have contact with discharged prisoners, though this varies from parole or mandatory post-release supervision schemes of the kind found in Australia, the Philippines and Britain to more marginal activities in Hungary and Israel.

Respondents were invited to comment on the *supervisory practice* of probation officers under three heads: counselling/casework, surveillance and social resource management. In all case study countries each is important, except in Western Australia where it is used only 'when identified as a need, so as to streamline services', counselling/casework is regarded as basic. Nevertheless there is confusion between counselling/casework and surveillance. In PNG for example, counselling/casework involves:

> patrolling rural areas and urban communities where offenders reside to see for themselves whether or not probationers are complying with court orders.

In South Australia counselling/casework has a temporal location as a diagnostic phase prior to the implementation of surveillance; in England and Wales where it is government policy to ground intervention in the 'principles of social work' the tension between the two is mentioned; and the New South Wales expert argues for a linking concept:

> Casework and surveillance are integral components of case management and are not seen as separate modes.

The various terms, however, are loose in meaning, umbrellas sheltering a range of tactical and strategic interventions conducted by the probation officer. In Scotland, probation workers:

are free to adopt those methods of work which they judge best suited to reducing the risk of further offending and assisting social integration.

In Hungary the expert observes:

Probation officers work individually; they have no set rules to follow about the modes of supervision.

Even in Israel, where the therapeutic orientation is well developed, the formulation is vague:

Suitable therapeutic and rehabilitation-oriented modes of supervision are applied to the offenders to modify their behaviour in the direction of the termination of criminal activity.

Japan offers an especially coherent formulation of the purpose of the activity but says nothing about the methods by which the purpose is pursued; only the very full Philippine response speaks of methods, offering a formulation of how the counselling/casework and surveillance modes interact, and how they in turn necessitate an acknowledgement of the social system of which offenders are a part:

Routine enquiries made by the probation officer during these interviews and also during home visits sometimes unearth adjustment problems which the offender must resolve either on his/her own, or which may need social intervention. ... The probation officer tends to look at the family, rather than the offender, as the unit of treatment, and this is aptly so since family ties in the Philippines are very strong and extend beyond the client's nuclear family. ... Group counselling and group-work are the more common modes of supervision practised in the rural areas. ... Resourceful probation officers use these occasions not only to discuss personal problems of their clients, but also to instruct them on such matters as civic duties, cleanliness and sanitation, or how to obtain credit or seek money for livelihood activities.

We enquired whether a belief existed that tensions between different aspects of the probation task led to *role strain or conflict*. With the exceptions of Israel and England and Wales respondents explained any such strain or conflict by the character of individual officers not by contradictions in probation itself. So in New South

Wales problems were experienced only by 'some' officers; in Japan by 'many'; in PNG there was 'minor confusion'; in the Philippines, though professional ideologies varied, a perception of care and control conflicting was rare; in Sweden and Scotland it was a problem only for some older officers who had failed to adjust to change. In England and Wales, however, the perception that strain or conflict existed was held by many; in Israel a structural rather than personal explanation was offered.

The historical accounts of probation provided in Part I illustrate the extent to which probation has to be perceived in terms of *social resource management*. Early common law probation officers found and exploited useful contacts closed to offenders, created training and employment opportunities, instilled regular habits by discouraging drinking and sought to heal any rifts between offenders and their social world which had resulted from the offence itself or from more generally negative social behaviour. As the Scottish expert put it:

> Offenders live in communities and the process of reconciliation which has to take place as a consequence of crime cannot happen without the community's involvement.

It is more in this area than in the 'private' one of individual supervision that we should expect obvious differences to emerge, since it is here that probation is most firmly rooted, organizationally, ideologically and economically, in its own 'locality'. In the largely Anglophone countries of Australia, Canada and Britain the trend, as in the USA, is away from a system of monopoly public service provision to a contract-based approach: responsibility for services remains with the state but the state's role involves purchasing as well as providing services. Hence in these countries the range of facilities developed to help, punish or monitor offenders emerges less from organic communities than from commercial systems whose continuation is measured in profitability not community support. In Canada:

> a probation officer will identify a particular problem or area in need of attention in an offender's case and will then seek out appropriate organizations in the community to fulfil that need.

In South Australia a range of specialist activities is subcontracted to agencies with specific skills and areas of involvement:

We advocate for the client and refer to other agency programmes including negotiations with accommodation agencies, drug and alcohol authorities, psychological or psychiatric assessment and/or treatment services, various other agencies such as child abuse, gambling, social security, unemployment, domestic violence, illiteracy and numeracy.

In the Philippines on the other hand, a less developed country, but one with a history and culture both of western colonialism and eastern tradition, probation is harnessed both to the crime itself and to national development goals. Hence it may involve programmes which are individualistically rehabilitative *and* designed to 'imbue [offenders] with a sense of nationhood and civic consciousness'. Offenders may accordingly be required to participate in activities geared to social/environmental improvement *or* to self-reliance and personal growth. So those guilty of illegally clearing forests for agriculture may be directed to forest conservation work to enable them to meet individualistic economic goals legally; while offenders convicted of illegal fishing or coral reef destruction may be trained in marine conservation and helped to buy fishing boats. Such activities co-exist, however, with counselling, an activity which is comprehensible both in terms of western colonialism and the Roman Catholic tradition of the Confession.

Nor can the use of *volunteers* be divorced from the broader social norms and relations of a given country. The more pretensions to western modes of expertise-driven professionalism probation officers have the more tensions are likely to emerge with volunteers. In Chapter 2 we noted the view of the clinically oriented officers of the 1950s that volunteers should be used only for financial reasons or because their 'enthusiasm might serve as a safeguard against administrative routine' (United Nations 1954a: 6); in many western countries volunteers are still viewed with circumspection by professionals, doubtless for job protection as well as professional reasons. Canada, Israel and Britain are, nonetheless, unusual in having no legislative basis for the use of volunteers and no central (as against local) policies for training, developing, supporting, supervising or managing them. That the framework for using volunteers in the very large and otherwise organizationally sophisticated probation service of England and Wales in particular is so weak in comparison to that which exists elsewhere in the world is a particularly striking finding of this study.

In the non-western societies of Japan, PNG and the Philippines, though they vary in duties, formal position and relations with professionals, volunteer probation officers are likely to emerge organically *from* the community. In the Philippines, with its centralized database of probation aides and more systematic programme of qualifications, training and support the position is nonetheless fairly formalized; in PNG it is less so:

> Volunteers who do not read nor write give verbal reports to the probation officer. . . . The VPO comes from the community the offender lives in. From talking and listening to the offender's family, close relatives and other influential community members the VPO becomes a catalyst in getting the community to support the probationer.

PROBATION ROUND THE WORLD

In this final section we highlight two key themes to have emerged from this study. While to create a typology of probation would be premature given our methodology and the lack of basic information about probation round the world on which the study could build, it is possible to identify issues which characterize probation practice as it has developed historically and as it is today.

We have made much of the *common and civil law origins* of probation – both how they are best comprehended as a product of the social, political and economic systems of which they are a part and how the framework of law itself constitutes a social product, comprising alongside other such products a public statement of the way a society is ordered. This social ordering can be grasped through dimensions such as colonialism, tribalism, urbanization, revolution and the social role of the churches, and we have tried to consider probation by interweaving these phenomena into the story we have to tell. Central to our approach, however, has been the position, articulated elsewhere, that the law is as much product as cause of social change:

> The wording, purpose and usage of law are, in this respect as in others, indistinguishable. Law is not the fount from which

social acts spring, but is itself a social product, and by no means necessarily the most influential.

(Harris and Timms 1993a: 21)

Not surprisingly therefore, as the social structures which created and sustained a particular 'type' of probation – reforming churchmen in the common, and revolutionary libertarian lawyers in the civil law tradition – began to dissolve, two processes began to occur. First there was a *convergence* between the common and civil law extremes so that the original bifurcation ceased to have meaning, and secondly a *transformation* within each which created new structures, but also new forms of restlessness.

Increasingly, therefore, common law countries came gradually to identify a vacuum in their penal arrangements which proba-tion, hitherto a 'floating' provision outside the sentencing structure, appeared well equipped to fill, albeit at the price of becoming less free, less dependent on the whim or personality of the supervising officer, and less variable in delivery. Conversely, in an acknowledgement of the practical limitations of rigid adher-ence to the principles of classical justice, most civil law countries had already begun to identify as a tactical inconvenience a restric-tiveness about probation which prevented it being exploited to solve those difficult cases where adherence to formula sentencing was patently inappropriate. And as these latter countries became receptive to a competing paradigm of criminal behaviour driven by the positive school of criminology, it became plausible for crime to be perceived not, or at least not solely, as a rational act, but as a symptom, beyond the grasp of the individual no doubt, but amenable to therapeutic expertise.

The dissemination of these ideas was facilitated by the steady growth of international congresses in late nineteenth-century Europe; the ideas contributed to the emergence of a form of supervision which was at first clinical and subsequently social in orientation, concerned less with the private reformation of the individual than with social rehabilitation into the community. In the ecological language of today this entailed creating a good-ness of fit between an individual's needs and the resources of the social world and, in the converse of this, between the repa-ration of the offender and the harm to the community caused by the criminal act. This latter theory, which elegantly served to legitimate a range of correctional activities such as community

service, conveniently married the urge to denounce with the urge
to repair.

In all this the probation service, its common and civil law
extremes having been softened into a more flexible arrangement,
was well placed to be helpful. Every act it was asked to perform
entailed both care and control, the resultant blurring being
reflected in our finding that counselling/casework and surveillance
were often used interchangeably.

These considerations make *volunteers and community involvement* crucial. The behaviour of many probationers is not easily
explicable or fitted into formalized sentencing structures. Such is
the complexity of the probation task that a unified notion of what
'constitutes' probation is by no means possible. In much probation round the world the blurring of care and control is further
complicated by a diversification of activity: as probation seeks by
varied means to hit a number of targets, volunteers and specialist
work supervisors contribute both to a more specialized division
of labour and a diversification of the labour itself.

In this move towards specialization the role of volunteers is
especially significant. Volunteers are *not* specialists but people
whose position *vis-à-vis* offenders reflects their social location
more generally. In Japan serving as a VPO both reflects and
augments one's social status, rather as serving as a lay magistrate
does in Great Britain; in Sweden and Papua New Guinea little
such status accrues and the use of volunteers reflects both cultural
norms and the practicalities of sparsely populated and (in the case
of PNG) hard to traverse countryside. In both countries the volunteer is from the offender's community and may be chosen on an
ad hoc basis to relate to the offender, not as part of a continuing
relationship with the probation service. In both countries the
offender may suggest a volunteer supervisor; in Sweden the status
of the volunteer is slightly confused by the fact that very modest
payment is made.

It is not entirely fanciful to see in the use of volunteers a recreation of the common law origins of probation itself (Harris 1992:
173). Volunteering entails law-abiding members of the community, with in most cases little by way of reward, training or status,
offering advice and support to those who have transgressed. The
social transformations associated with early industrialization led
to the marginalization and personal dislocation of numerous
vulnerable people whose petty criminality brought them to the

attention of strangers, not as hitherto to less formal and more localized control systems. Accordingly relatively primitive (though ostensibly very scientific) sanctions were at this time exercised in a manner unmediated by the flexibility which stems from prior knowledge. The emphasis on 'relationship' in much probation work, however, provided just such prior knowledge, creating at times an emotional identification which encompassed officer and offender alike. Few early probation officers, having heard a probationer's tale, can have failed at some time to think 'there but for the grace of God go I'; so while the knowledge which stemmed from talking provided – as knowledge always does – a new technology of power to be mediated by the officer, it provided too, and equally ubiquitously[3] a compassionate understanding which paved the way for a tactical flexibility in the work of the pioneer British and American probation officers. It was this flexibility which so impressed the countries whose probation tradition lay in the *sursis*.

Nevertheless the transformations in probation of the late twentieth century – not only in Australia, Canada, Britain and the USA but also in Sweden and elsewhere in Western Europe – have moved common law probation in the direction of sanction as a means of tackling the policy problem of an excess of prison numbers at a time of rising crime. Even in Scotland, where probation has long been located in social work departments, changes consistent with trends elsewhere have been wrought by a funding change:

> Scotland has witnessed, over the past four to five years, the most significant developments in the provision of social work services to offenders and their families since the disbanding of the probation service and the creation of generic social work departments in 1969. The introduction of full central government funding has undoubtedly provided a much-needed impetus to the development of statutory services to the criminal justice system. ... The price of the new arrangements is, however, increased accountability and centralized control.
>
> (McIvor 1994: 443)

This trend in turn creates a new void, as those who pose fewer problems through their criminal behaviour than they experience as human beings, whom no one especially wants to punish more than is necessary to mark the wrongness of their acts but whose need for support to get through life unscathed is manifest, become excluded from the new arrangements. When, as is inevitable given the rise of probation round the world, the costs of probation become of such political significance that formal supervision of minor offenders is rated uneconomic, supervision by a volunteer seems wholly sensible, particularly if the volunteer is from the community into which the offender is to be reintegrated.

The case study countries considered in this book exist at different points on a multiplex of continua. One continuum – of *professionalization* – places the economically stretched and nascent Hungarian and PNG services at one extreme and the highly professionalized orientation of Israel at the other. Another scale, between *treatment and control*, places Israel again at one extreme but the former common law countries of Australia, Canada and (increasingly) England and Wales at the other. In terms of *size* the services vary between the massive English and Welsh service (12,000 full-time equivalent personnel) and PNG (88) or Hungary (100). In terms of *community involvement* Japan, Sweden and PNG have an excess of volunteers over probation officers, whereas at the other extreme Israel makes no significant use of volunteers at all; while in spite of having one of the largest and most systematically organized probation systems in the world, England and Wales has no centrally available information as to the numbers of volunteers. It is doubtless significant that both the Israeli and the English and Welsh probation services are highly professionalized and unionized.

Many more axes could be constructed and doubtless will be in future work. When they are it is recommended that they be augmented by qualitative information of a kind our methods have not enabled us to secure. Our aim has been more modest: to chart what we know of the development and present character of probation generally, and to draw on work undertaken in the case study countries to give an idea of both the diversity of probation round the world and of what commonalities underpin such diversity. These commonalities include the relation of probation to law and culture, and to social organization and structure; they are reflected in the belief that to aim to change offenders for the better is a proper function for a criminal justice system, and that probation supervision can help it perform this function.

Underpinning much of this book is a concern to discourage reification and essentialism by stressing that probation is not a 'thing' to be taken or left but a set of ideas and possibilities to be used creatively and strategically to solve local problems of criminal justice. This is a point of practical as well as analytic significance. Given that some readers may be policy makers in developing countries wishing to introduce probation, our message is that probation is not an external solution to internal problems of criminal justice or penology, but a possible framework into which locally feasible and desirable solutions may be fitted.

This is not to deny, however, that to develop a probation system has economic, political and professional implications; nor is it to deny that much learning is available from the history of probation. This learning advises, first and negatively, against developing a strong therapeutic orientation: therapeutic modes of probation have high costs in terms of staff training (which will almost certainly be overseas); what we know of their effectiveness in reducing crime is not encouraging; nor have they always been successfully imported from the west, and they may, as in India, offer a false dawn which obscures the real needs of the criminal justice system there: to promote literacy, rural development, racial and religious harmony and the successful reintegration of offenders into rejecting communities. Nor should it be forgotten that most western countries have abandoned psychoanalytically derived therapy as a way forward.

If probation is to prosper in developing countries it must build on existing structures of social support by working to enhance what is already there and repairing any fractures to the social fabric brought about by rapid social change. It is sensible to begin by means of functional analysis: explore what modes of non-custodial punishment are desirable, why they are desirable, what they are intended to achieve, and how. It is advisable to involve members of the community, not necessarily only on the individualistic basis of western volunteering but possibly drawing too on the former Eastern European tradition which sees supervision as by and in the community. Though reliability and probity are necessary for supervisors, high levels of clinical skill are not, a fact which may be as pertinent to those highly qualified western probation services which have been reluctant to exploit the use and availability of volunteers as for policy makers in the developing world. Where supervision is by the community, probation becomes a legal framework to differentiate supervision from friendship and support, and to mark it out as a disposition of the court which when discharged demonstrates that the offender's debt has been paid.

There are other changes discernible in probation round the world. There is in most countries a greater emphasis on account-ability, firmness of resolve and clarity of purpose; and probation today is often not a single sentence but a framework for community corrections, containing the possibility of combinations of sentence, gradated according to the gravity of the crime or the circumstances of the criminal. This has come about partly epiphe-nomenally, as a by-product of political moves to the right which have characterized many western democracies since the early 1980s; but its roots go deeper, showing that as probation has matured there is greater appreciation of its strategic potential and of the necessity of a combination of flexibility and relevance in criminal justice. Hence the convergence of the common and civil law traditions: to be of greatest value probation must combine flexibility with system centrality; common law probation can offer the former but not the latter; civil law probation can offer the latter without the former. Neither paradigm is a helpful way forward today.

In the abandonment of the *a priori* principles embodied in common or civil law, however, a new character of probation has emerged which ensures that it addresses in a practical way local social and criminal concerns. These may include the overuse of prison, an undesirable reliance on physical punishment, the problems of juvenile offenders, the rehabilitation of criminals or reparation for victims. Probation acknowledges that no criminal justice system, however sophisticated, can deal definitively at the point of sentence with every hard case which comes its way. As a flexible resource to solve such problems, to monitor progress in doubtful cases or to suggest a way forward where normal disposals are inappropriate, probation can be moulded in any way which will be helpful. A book such as this can provide information from which ideas can emerge. Of these some will doubtless be discarded, others may be worth consideration. To provide a general blueprint for probation where no probation exists, however, is impossible. A book about probation round the world may raise more questions than it can give answers;

to answer local questions, however, is the job of local policy makers not comparative researchers.

NOTES

1 In particular, quotations are taken from raw data provided by the experts as a basis for Part II, and not necessarily from Part II itself. In a few cases minor amendments have been made to the wording in order to improve clarity of expression.
2 Two further points are worthy of mention about the Israeli service: it has one of the highest proportions of female officers (only Sweden in our study has more while Japan and PNG have almost none) and the highest proportion of professional staff in the workforce.
3 The French aphorism *tout comprendre, c'est tout pardonner* is, in this context, perceptive if slightly hyperbolic.

Bibliography

Abadinsky, H. (1991) *Probation and Parole: Theory and Practice*. 4th Ed. Englewood Cliffs, NJ: Prentice-Hall.

Allen, G. (1987) 'Where are We Going in Criminal Justice? Some Insights from the Chinese Criminal Justice System'. *International Journal of Offender Therapy and Comparative Criminology*. 31, 101–110.

Allen, H. and Simonsen, C. (1978) *Corrections in America: an Introduction*. 2nd Ed. Encino, CA: Collier Macmillan.

Allen, H., Eskridge, C., Latessa, E. and Vito, G. (1985) *Probation and Parole in America*. New York: Free Press.

Alvazzi del Frate, A., Zvekic, U. and van Dijk, J. (eds) (1993) *Understanding Crime: Experiences of Crime and Crime Control*. Rome: United Nations Interregional Crime and Justice Research Institute.

Ancel, M. (1971) *Suspended Sentence*. London: Heinemann Educational Books.

Armer, M. (1973) 'Methodological Problems and Possibilities in Comparative Research'. In M. Armer and A. Grimshaw op. cit.

Armer, M. and Grimshaw, A. (eds) (1973) *Comparative Social Research: Methodological Problems and Strategies*. New York: John Wiley.

Armstrong, T. (ed.) (1991) *Intensive Interventions with High-Risk Youths: Promising Approaches in Juvenile Probation and Parole*. Monsey, NY: Criminal Justice Press.

Ayscough, H. (1923) *When Mercy Seasons Justice: a Short History of the Work of the Church of England in the Police Courts*. Westminster: Church of England Temperance Society.

Balfour, J. (1907) *My Prison Life*. London: Chapman and Hall.

Bartollas, C. (1985) *Correctional Treatment: Theory and Practice*. Englewood Cliffs, NJ: Prentice-Hall.

Bensinger, G. (1982) 'Criminal Justice in Israel'. *Journal of Criminal Justice*. 10, 393–401.

Bensinger, G. (1984) 'Corrections in Israel and the United States: a Comparative Analysis'. *International Journal of Comparative and Applied Criminal Justice*. 8, 55–62.

Berting, J. (1988) 'Research Strategies in International Comparative and Cooperative Research: the Case of the Vienna Centre'. In F. Charvat,

W. Stamatiou and Ch. Villain-Gandossi op. cit.

Bhattacharyya, S. (1980) 'Organisational Pattern of Probation Services, Methods of Recruitment and Training in Britain and India: a Comparative Study'. *Social Defence*. 16, 5–16.

Bhattacharyya, S. (1986) *Probation System in India: an Appraisal*. Delhi: Manas Publications.

Bien, T., Miller, W. and Tonigan, J. (1993) 'Brief Interventions for Alcohol Problems: a Review'. *Addiction*. 88, 315–336.

Blomberg, T. and Lucken, K. (1994) 'Stacking the Deck by Piling up Sanctions? Is Intermediate Punishment Destined to Fail?' *Howard Journal of Criminal Justice*. 33, 62–80.

Blos, P. (1962) *On Adolescence: a Psychoanalytic Interpretation*. New York: Free Press.

Bochel, D. (1976) *Probation and After-Care: Its Development in England and Wales*. Edinburgh: Scottish Academic Press.

Booth, C. (1890) *In Darkest England and the Way Out*. London: Salvation Army.

Braithwaite, J. (1989) *Crime, Shame and Reintegration*. Cambridge: Cambridge University Press.

Breda, R. and Ferracuti, F. (1980) 'Alternatives to Incarceration in Italy'. *Crime and Delinquency*. 26, 63–69.

Brillon, Y. (1980) *Ethnocriminology of Black Africa*. Montréal: Presses de l'Université de Montréal.

Brown, P. (1990) 'Guns and Probation Officers: the Unspoken Reality'. *Federal Probation*. LII, 21–25.

Brownlee, I. and Joanes, D. (1993) 'Intensive Probation for Young Adult Offenders: Evaluating the Impact of a Non-Custodial Sentence'. *British Journal of Criminology*. 33, 216–230.

Brydensholt, H. (1980) 'Crime Policy in Denmark: How we Managed to Reduce the Prison Population'. *Crime and Delinquency*. 26, 35–41.

Byrne, J. (1990) 'The Future of Intensive Probation Supervision and the New Intermediate Sanctions'. *Crime and Delinquency*. 36, 238–256.

Byrne, J., Lurigio, A. and Baird, C. (1989) 'The Effectiveness of the New Intensive Supervision Programs'. *Research in Corrections*. 2, 1–48.

Carpenter, M. (1851) *Reformatory Schools for the Children of the Perishing and Dangerous Classes and for Juvenile Delinquents*. London: Gilpin.

Carter, R. and Wilkins, L. (eds) (1970) *Probation and Parole: Selected Readings*. New York: John Wiley.

Cartledge, C., Tak, P. and Tomic-Malic, M. (eds) (1981) *Probation in/en Europe*. Hertogenbosch, Netherlands: European Assembly for Probation and After Care.

Chakrabarti, N. (1992) 'Is Rehabilitation Essential in the Probation Service in West Bengal?' *International Journal of Offender Therapy and Comparative Criminology*. 36, 121–128.

Chappell, D. and Wilson, P. (eds) (1986) *The Australian Criminal Justice System: the Mid-1980s*. Sydney: Butterworth.

Charvat, F., Stamatiou, W. and Villain-Gandossi, Ch. (eds) (1988) *International Cooperation in the Social Sciences: 25 Years of Vienna*

Centre Experience. Bratislava: Publishing House of the Technical Library.

Chute, C. and Bell, M. (1956) *Crime, Courts and Probation*. New York: Macmillan.

Clear, T. and Cole, G. (1986) *American Corrections*. Monterey, CA: Brooks/Cole.

Clear, T. and O'Leary, V. (1983) *Controlling the Offender in the Community*. Lexington, MA: D.C. Heath.

Clear, T. and Rumgay, J. (1992) 'Divided by a Common Language: British and American Probation Cultures'. *Federal Probation*. LVI, 3–11.

Clifford, W. (1974) *Introduction to African Criminology*. Nairobi: Oxford University Press.

Clifford, W. (ed.) (1980) *Corrections in Asia and the Pacific*. Canberra: Australian Institute of Criminology.

Clifford, W. (ed.) (1983) *The Management of Corrections in Asia and the Pacific: Proceedings of the Third Asian and Pacific Conference of Correctional Administrators*. Canberra: Australian Institute of Criminology.

Cohen, B.-Z., Eden, R. and Lazar, A. (1991) 'The Efficacy of Probation versus Imprisonment in Reducing Recidivism of Serious Offenders in Israel'. *Journal of Criminal Justice*. 19, 263–270.

Cohen, S. (1982) 'Western Crime Control Models in the Third World: Benign or Malignant?' In S. Spitzer and R. Simon op. cit.

Cohen, S. (1985) *Visions of Social Control: Crime, Punishment and Classification*. Cambridge: Polity Press.

Cole, G., Frankowski, S. and Gertz, M. (eds) (1987) *Major Criminal Justice Systems*. London: Sage.

Conférence Permanente Européenne de la Probation (1983) *Alternative Ways in Dealing with Delinquent Behaviour: Report of the General Assembly*. Hertogenbosch, Netherlands: Algemene Reclasseringsvereninging.

Council of Europe (1970) *Practical Organisation of Measures for the Supervision and After-Care of Conditionally Sentenced or Conditionally Released Offenders: Report of the European Committee on Crime Problems*. Strasbourg: Council of Europe.

Croft, J. (1979) *Crime and Comparative Research*. Home Office Research Study No. 57. London: HMSO.

Davies, M. (1989) *Probation Reading: an Empirical Bibliography*. Norwich, University of East Anglia: Social Work Monographs.

Day, S. (1858) *Juvenile Crime, its Causes, Character and Cure*. London: J.F. Hope.

Department of Correctional Services (South Australia) (1987) *Home Detention*. DI No. 105 (unpublished mimeograph). Adelaide: Government of South Australia.

Diana, L. (1970) 'What is Probation?' In R. Carter and L. Wilkins op. cit.

Donzelot, J. (1980) *The Policing of Families: Welfare Versus the State*. London: Hutchinson.

Downes, D. (1982) 'The Origins and Consequences of Dutch Penal Policy

Since 1945: a Preliminary Analysis'. *British Journal of Criminology.* 22, 325–342.

Downes, D. (1988) *Contrasts in Tolerance: Post-War Penal Policy in the Netherlands and England and Wales.* Oxford: The Clarendon Press.

Drakeford, M. (1993) 'The Probation Service, Breach and the Criminal Justice Act 1991'. *Howard Journal of Criminal Justice.* 32, 291–303.

Dressler, D. (1969) *Practice and Theory of Probation and Parole.* 2nd Ed. New York: Columbia University Press.

Durst, D. (1992) 'The Road to Poverty is Paved with Good Intentions: Social Interventions and Indigenous Peoples'. *International Social Work.* 35, 191–202.

Edholm, L. and Bishop, N. (1983) *Serious Drug Misusers in the Swedish Prison and Probation System.* Norrkoeping: Sweden National Prison and Probation Administration.

Eggleston, E. (1976) *Fear, Favour or Affection – Aborigines and the Criminal Law in Victoria, South Australia and Western Australia.* Canberra: Australian National University Press.

Ekstedt, J. and Griffiths, C. (1988) *Corrections in Canada.* Toronto: Butterworth.

Elder, J. (1973) 'Problems of Cross-Cultural Methodology: Instrumentation and Interviewing in India'. In M. Armer and A. Grimshaw op. cit.

Eskridge, C. and Newbold, G. (1993) 'Corrections in New Zealand'. *Federal Probation.* 57, 59–66.

Falkowski-Tucker, T. (1990) 'Starting Over: Developing a Probation Service in the East of Germany'. *Probation Journal.* 37, 182–185.

Farrington, D. and Walklate, S. (eds) (1993) *Offenders and Victims: Theory and Policy. British Criminology Conference 1991: Selected Papers Volume 1.* London: British Society of Criminology in association with the Institute for the Study and Treatment of Delinquency.

Faulkner, D. (1989) 'The Future of the Probation Service: a View from Government'. In R. Shaw and K. Haines op. cit.

Fauteux Commission (1956) *Report of a Committee Appointed to Inquire into the Principles and Procedures Followed in the Remission Service of the Department of Justice of Canada.* Ottawa: Department of Justice.

Fielder, M. (1992) 'Purchasing and Providing Services for Offenders: Lessons from America'. In R. Statham and P. Whitehead op. cit.

Fielding, N. (1984) *Probation Practice: Client Support Under Social Control.* Aldershot: Gower.

Findlay, M. and Zvekic, U. (1988) *Analysing (In)formal Mechanisms of Crime Control: a Cross-Cultural Perspective.* Rome: United Nations Social Defence Research Institute.

Findlay, M. and Zvekic, U. (1993) *Alternative Policing Styles: Cross-Cultural Perspectives.* Deventer: Kluwer.

Fink, A. (1938) *Causes of Crime: Biological Theories in the United States 1800–1915.* Philadelphia: University of Pennsylvania Press.

Finn, P. and Parent, D. (1993) 'Texas Collects Substantial Revenues from Probation Fees'. *Federal Probation.* LVII, 17–22.

Finsterbusch, K. (1973) 'The Sociology of Nation-States: Dimensions, Indicators, and Theory'. In M. Armer and A. Grimshaw op. cit.

Fitzpatrick, P. (1982) 'The Political Economy of Dispute Settlement in Papua New Guinea'. In C. Sumner op. cit.

Fogel, D. (1984) 'The Emergence of Probation as a Profession in the Service of Public Safety: the Next Ten Years'. In P. McAnany, D. Thomson and D. Fogel op. cit.

Form, W. (1973) 'Field Problems in Comparative Research: the Politics of Distrust'. In M. Armer and A. Grimshaw op. cit.

Forsythe, W. (1987) The Reform of Prisoners 1830–1900. London: Croom Helm.

Forsythe, W. (1993) 'Women Prisoners and Women Penal Officials 1840–1921'. British Journal of Criminology. 33, 525–540.

Foucault, M. (1977) Discipline and Punish: the Birth of the Prison. (Trans. Alan Sheridan). Harmondsworth: Allen Lane.

Fox, L. (1952) The English Prison and Borstal Systems. London: Routledge and Kegan Paul.

Freud, A. (1937) The Ego and the Mechanisms of Defence. London: Hogarth Press.

Friedlander, K. (1947) The Psychoanalytic Approach to Juvenile Delinquency. London: Kegan Paul, Trench, Trubner and Company.

Frishtik, M. (1988) 'The Probation Officer's Recommendation in his "Investigation Report" '. Journal of Offender Counselling, Services and Rehabilitation. 13, 101–132.

Frishtik, M. (1991) 'The Sentencing of Young Adult Offenders in Israeli Courts: Punishment versus Imprisonment'. Journal of Criminal Justice. 19, 525–536.

Gale, F., Bailey-Harris, R. and Wundersitz, J. (1991) Aboriginal Youth and the Criminal Justice System: the Injustice of Justice. Oakleigh, Victoria: Cambridge University Press.

Glover, E. (1949) Probation and Re-Education. London: Routledge and Kegan Paul.

Gordon, M. (1976) Involving Paraprofessionals in the Helping Process: the Case of Federal Probation. Cambridge, MA: Ballinger.

Greenwood, P. with Abrahamse, A. (1982) Selective Incapacitation. Prepared for the National Department of Justice, US Department of Justice. Santa Monica, CA: Rand Corporation.

Grimshaw, A. (1973) 'Comparative Sociology: in What Ways Different from Other Sociologies?' In M. Armer and A. Grimshaw op. cit.

Grünhut, M. (1948) Penal Reform: a Comparative Study. Oxford: The Clarendon Press.

Grünhut, M. (1952) 'Probation in Germany'. Howard Journal of Criminal Justice. VIII, 168–173.

Grünhut, M. (1956) Juvenile Offenders Before the Courts. Oxford: The Clarendon Press.

Grünhut, M. (1963) Probation and Mental Treatment. London: Tavistock Publications.

Gumperz, J. (1971) Language in Social Groups: Essays by John J. Gumperz. Selected and Introduced by A. Dil. Stanford, CA:

Stanford University Press.

Hackler, J. and Brockman, J. (1980) 'Opinion-Role Typologies for Cross-Cultural Comparisons of Juvenile Courts'. *Juvenile and Family Court Journal*. 31, 61–76.

Hall, E. (1966) *The Hidden Dimension*. New York: Doubleday.

Harris, R. (1989a) *Suffer the Children, the Family, the State and the Social Worker*. Inaugural Lecture. Hull: Hull University Press.

Harris, R. (1989b) 'Social Work in Society or Punishment in the Community?' In R. Shaw and K. Haines op. cit.

Harris, R. (1992) *Crime, Criminal Justice and the Probation Service*. London: Routledge.

Harris, R. (1994) 'Continuity and Change: Probation and Politics in Contemporary Britain'. *International Journal of Offender Therapy and Comparative Criminology*. 38, 33–45.

Harris, R. (1995) 'Child Protection, Child Care and Child Welfare'. In K. Wilson and A. James op. cit.

Harris, R. and Timms, N. (1993a) *Secure Accommodation and Child Care: Between Hospital and Prison or Thereabouts*. London: Routledge.

Harris, R. and Timms, N. (1993b) 'The Lost Key: Secure Accommodation and Juvenile Crime: an English and Welsh Perspective'. *Australian and New Zealand Journal of Criminology*. 26(3), 219–231.

Harris, R. and Webb, D. (1987) *Welfare, Power and Juvenile Justice: the Social Control of Delinquent Youth*. London: Tavistock Publications.

Hatt, K. (1985) 'Probation and Corrections in a Neo-Correctional Era'. *Canadian Journal of Criminology*. 27, 299–316.

Haxby, D. (1978) *Probation: a Changing Service*. London: Constable.

Heidensohn, F. and Farrell, M. (eds) (1991) *Crime in Europe*. London: Routledge.

Heijder, A. (1967) 'Some Characteristics of the Dutch Probation System'. *International Journal of Offender Therapy*. 11, 89–93.

Heijder, A. (1972) 'Some Aspects of the Dutch Probation System: a Search for Identity'. *International Journal of Offender Therapy and Comparative Criminology*. 17, 106–110.

Heiland, H.-G., Shelley, L. and Katoh, H. (eds) (1991) *Crime and Control in Comparative Perspectives*. Berlin: de Gruyter.

Henkel, M. (1991a) *Government, Evaluation and Change*. London: Jessica Kingsley.

Henkel, M. (1991b) 'The New "Evaluative State"'. *Public Administration*. 69, 121–136.

Hess, A. (1970) 'The Volunteer Probation Officers of Japan'. *International Journal of Offender Therapy*. 14, 8–14.

Hink, H. (1962) 'The Application of Constitutional Standards of Protection to Probation'. *The University of Chicago Law Review*. 29, 483–497.

Hobhouse, L., Wheeler, G. and Ginsberg, M. (1930) *The Material Culture and Social Institutions of the Simpler Peoples: an Essay in Correlation*. London: Chapman and Hall.

Hogan, M. (1971) 'Probation in Japan'. *Probation*. 17, 8–11.

Holmes, T. (1900) *Pictures and Problems from London Police Courts*. London: Edward Arnold.

Holt, R. and Turner, J. (eds) (1970) *The Methodology of Comparative Research*. New York: Free Press.

Home Office (1956) 'Probation Today and Tomorrow: Notes from the Probation Division of the Home Office'. *Howard Journal of Criminal Justice*. IX, 245–249.

Home Office (1993) *PTU Strategy: Draft 11/93*. Probation Training Unit: Mimeographed Working Document. London: Home Office.

Honderich, T. (1969) *Punishment: the Supposed Justifications*. London: Hutchinson.

Hood, R. (1989) *The Death Penalty: a World-Wide Perspective*. Oxford: Oxford University Press.

Hope, D. (1988) *The Relation of Aboriginal Customary Law to the General Law*. Mimeograph. Adelaide: Report to the Justice and Consumer Affairs Committee of Cabinet, on behalf of the Task Force on Aboriginals and Criminal Justice.

Hudson, B. (1993) *Penal Policy and Social Justice*. London: Macmillan.

Hylton, J. (1981) 'The Growth of Punishment: Imprisonment and Community Corrections in Canada'. *Crime and Social Justice*. 15, 18–28.

Hymes, D. (1970) 'Linguistic Aspects of Comparative Political Research'. In R. Holt and J. Turner op. cit.

Igbinovia, P. (1989) 'Criminology in Africa'. *International Journal of Offender Therapy and Comparative Criminology*. 33, v–x.

Jeyasingh, J. (1982) 'Problems in the Practice of Probation: the Indian Experience'. *Indian Journal of Criminology and Criminalistics*. 2, 202–205.

Junger-Tas, J. and Tigges, L. (1982) *Probation, After-Care, Child-Care and Protection*. The Hague: Ministry of Justice.

Kaplan, A. (1964) *The Conduct of Inquiry: Methodology for Social Research*. San Francisco: Chandler.

Karmen, A. (1980) 'Race, Inferiority, Crime and Research Taboos'. In E. Sagarin op. cit.

Keefe, W. (1972) 'The Adult Probation Authority in New South Wales'. *International Journal of Offender Therapy and Comparative Criminology*. 17, 83–89.

Keris, P. (1989) *Annual Report for 1988*. Department of Attorney-General Village Courts Secretariat. Waigani, PNG: Central Government Offices.

Keris, P. (1992) *Information Paper on Papua New Guinea Village Courts System*. Department of Attorney-General Village Courts Secretariat. Waigani, PNG: Central Government Offices.

King, J. (ed.) (1958) *The Probation Service*. London: Butterworth.

Klein, M. (ed.) (1984) *Western Systems of Juvenile Justice*. Beverly Hills, CA: Sage.

Kohn, M. (ed.) (1989a) *Cross-National Research in Sociology*. Newbury Park, CA: Sage.

Kohn, M. (1989b) 'Cross-National Research as an Analytic Strategy'. In M. Kohn op. cit.

Kohn, M. (1989c) 'Introduction'. In M. Kohn op. cit.

Lee, Sun-Man (1972) 'The Probation Service in Hong Kong'. *International Journal of Offender Therapy and Comparative Criminology.* 17, 90–94.

Leivesley, S. (1986) 'Alternatives to Imprisonment'. In D. Chappell and P. Wilson op. cit.

Lemert, E. (1993) 'Visions of Social Control: Probation Reconsidered'. *Crime and Delinquency.* 39, 447–461.

Le Mesurier, L. (1935) *A Handbook of Probation and Social Work of the Courts.* London: National Association of Probation Officers.

Lindner, C. (1992) 'The Refocused Home Visit: a Subtle but Revolutionary Change'. *Federal Probation.* LVI, 16–21.

Lindner, C. and Koehler, R. (1992) 'Probation Officer Victimization: an Emerging Concern'. *Journal of Criminal Justice.* 20, 53–62.

Locke, T. (1990) *New Approaches to Crime in the 1990s: Planning Responses to Crime.* London: Longman.

López–Rey, M. (1957) 'United Nations Activities and International Trends in Probation'. *Howard Journal of Penal Policy.* 9, 346–353.

López-Rey, M. (1976) 'United Nations Policy in Crime Problems – the Problem of Crime and the Problem of Criminology'. *International Journal of Criminology and Penology.* 4, 59–67.

Lorenz, W. (1994) *Social Work in a Changing Europe.* London: Routledge.

McAnany, P., Thomson, D. and Fogel, D. (eds) (1984) *Probation and Justice: Reconsideration of Mission.* Cambridge, MA: Oelgeschlager, Gunn and Hain.

McBean, J. (1972) 'Probation in Jamaica'. *International Journal of Offender Therapy and Comparative Criminology.* 17, 95–105.

McCarthy, B. (1987) *Intermediate Punishment: Intensive Supervision, Home Confinement and Electronic Monitoring.* Monsey, NY: Criminal Justice Press.

McCarthy, B. and McCarthy Jr, B. (1991) *Community Based Corrections.* 2nd Ed. Pacific Grove, CA: Brooks/Cole.

McGuire, J. and Priestley, P. (1985) *Offending Behaviour: Skills and Stratagems for Going Straight.* London: Batsford.

McIvor, G. (1994) 'Social Work and Criminal Justice in Scotland: Developments in Policy and Practice'. *British Journal of Social Work.* 24, 429–448.

McWilliams, W. (1983) 'The Mission to the English Police Courts 1876–1936'. *Howard Journal of Penology and Crime Prevention.* XXII, 129–147.

Mair, G. and Nee, C. (1990) *Electronic Monitoring: the Trials and their Results.* Home Office Research Study No. 120. London: HMSO.

Mandal, K. (1989) 'American Influence on Social Work Education in India and its Impact'. *International Social Work.* 32, 303–309.

Martinson, R. (1974) 'What Works? Questions and Answers about Prison Reform'. *The Public Interest.* 35, 22–54.

Mawby, R. (1990) *Comparative Policing Issues: the British and American Experience in International Perspective.* London: Routledge.

May, T. (1991) *Probation: Politics, Policy and Practice*. Milton Keynes: Open University Press.

Meyer, P. (1983) *The Child and the State: The Intervention of the State in Family Life*. (Trans. J. Ennew and J. Lloyd). Cambridge and Paris: Cambridge University Press and Editions de la Maison des Sciences de l'Homme.

Midgley, J. (1977) 'Crime in South Africa: a Comparative Analysis'. *South African Journal of Criminal Law and Criminology*. 1, 71–92.

Milner, A. (1972) *The Nigerian Penal System*. London: Sweet and Maxwell.

Monger, M. (1964) *Casework in Probation*. London: Butterworth.

Moriyama, T. (1989) 'Informal Mechanism of Crime Control in Japan'. *Journal of Takusho University*. 178, 17–37.

Morris, N. and Tonry, M. (1990) *Between Prison and Probation: Intermediate Punishments in a Rational Sentencing System*. New York: Oxford University Press.

Moxon, D. (ed.) (1985) *Managing Criminal Justice: a Collection of Papers*. London: HMSO.

Mushanga, T. (ed.) (1992) *Criminology in Africa*. UNICRI Series Criminology in Developing Countries. Rome: United Nations Interregional Crime and Justice Research Institute.

Nagpaul, H. (1993) 'Analysis of Social Work Teaching Material in India: the Need for Indigenous Foundations'. *International Social Work*. 36, 207–220.

Nakayama, K. (1987) 'Japan'. In G. Cole, S. Frankowski and M. Gertz op. cit.

Nalla, M. and Newman, G. (1991) 'The Sentencing of Young Adult Offenders in Israeli Courts: Probation versus Imprisonment'. *Journal of Criminal Justice*. 19, 525–536.

National Institute of Mental Health (1971) *Crime and Delinquency Research in Selected European Countries*. Crime and Delinquency Topics: a Monograph Series. Rockville, MD: National Institute of Mental Health Center for Studies of Crime and Delinquency.

Nelson, A. (1987) 'Sweden'. In G. Cole, S. Frankowski and M. Gertz op. cit.

Nishikawa, M. (1994) 'Adult Probation in Japan'. In U. Zvekic op. cit.

Noonan, S. and Latessa, E. (1987) 'Intensive Probation: an Examination of Recidivism and Social Adjustment for an Intensive Supervision Program'. *American Journal of Criminal Justice*. 12, 45–61.

Nuyten-Edelbroek, E. and Tigges, L. (1980) 'Early Intervention in a Probation Agency: a Netherlands Experiment'. *Howard Journal of Criminal Justice*. XIX, 42-51.

Nyquist, O. (1960) *Juvenile Justice: a Comparative Study with Special Reference to the Swedish Child Welfare Board and the California Juvenile Court System*. London: Macmillan.

Oommen, T. (1989) 'Ethnicity, Immigration, and Cultural Pluralism: India and the United States of America'. In M. Kohn op. cit.

Øyen, E. (ed.) (1990) *Comparative Methodology: Theory and Practice in International Social Research*. Newbury Park, CA: Sage.

Page, M. (1992) *Crimefighters of London: a History of the Origins and Development of the London Probation Service 1876–1965*. London: Inner London Probation Service Benevolent and Educational Trust.

Paliwala, A. (1982) 'Law and Order in the Village: Papua New Guinea's Village Courts'. In C. Sumner op. cit.

Parsloe, P. (1969) 'Probation in Britain: Factors Influencing the Probation Officer's Choice of Work with Clients'. *International Journal of Offender Therapy*. 13, 91–99.

Parton, N. (1985) *The Politics of Child Abuse*. London: Macmillan Education.

Paternoster, R. and Bynum, T. (1982) 'The Justice Model as Ideology: a Critical Look at the Impetus for Sentencing Reform'. *Contemporary Crises*. 6, 7–24.

Pelikan, C. (1991) 'Conflict Resolution Between Victims and Offenders in Austria and the Federal Republic of Germany'. In F. Heidensohn and M. Farrell op. cit.

Petersilia, J. (1987) 'Probation and Felony Offenders'. *Federal Probation*. LI, 56–61.

Petersilia, J. and Turner, S. (1991) *Intensive Supervision for High Risk Probationers*. Santa Monica, CA: Rand Corporation.

Petersilia, J., Turner, S., Kahan, J. and Peterson, J. (1985) *Granting Felons Probation*. Santa Monica, CA: Rand Corporation.

Platt, A. (1969) *The Child Savers: the Invention of Delinquency*. Chicago: University of Chicago Press.

Portes, A. (1973) 'Perception of the US Sociologist and its Impact on Cross-National Research'. In M. Armer and A. Grimshaw op. cit.

Pound, R. (1975) *Criminal Justice in America*. New York: Da Capo Press. (Originally published by Brown University Press, 1930.)

Pratt, J. (1990) 'The Future of the Probation Service in New Zealand'. *The Australian and New Zealand Journal of Criminology*. 23, 105–116.

Priestley, P. (1985) *Victorian Prison Lives: English Prison Biography 1830–1914*. London: Methuen.

Ragin, C. (1989) 'New Directions in Comparative Research'. In M. Kohn op. cit.

Raynor, P. (1978) 'Compulsory Persuasion: a Problem for Correctional Social Work'. *British Journal of Social Work*. 8, 411–424.

Raynor, P. (1985) *Social Work, Justice and Control*. Oxford: Basil Blackwell.

Rehabilitation Bureau, Ministry of Justice, Japan (1990) *Community-Based Treatment of Offenders in Japan*. Tokyo: Ministry of Justice.

Reid, W. and Shyne, A. (1970) *Brief and Extended Casework*. New York: Columbia University Press.

Reifen, D. (1969) 'Probation in Israel: the Legal Background'. *International Journal of Offender Therapy*. 13, 106–110.

Report from the Departmental Committee on Prisons (1895) Cmnd 7702 (Gladstone Report).

Report of the Departmental Committee on the Probation Service (1962) Cmnd 1650 (Morison Report).

Rodenborg, N. (1986) 'A Western-Style Counselling Office in Somalia:

a Case Study of Cultural Conflicts in Social Work Practice'. *International Social Work*. 29, 43–55.

Rose, G. (1967) *Schools for Young Offenders*. London: Tavistock Publications.

Ross, R.R. and Fabiano, E.A. (1985) *Time to Think: a Cognitive Model of Delinquency Prevention and Rehabilitation*. Ottawa: Institute of Social Sciences and Arts.

Ross, R.R., Fabiano, E.A. and Ewles, C.D. (1988) 'Reasoning and Rehabilitation'. *International Journal of Offender Therapy and Comparative Criminology*. 20, 165–173.

Rotimi, A. and Oloruntimehin, O. (1992) 'Teaching and Research Network in Africa in the Field of Criminology'. In T. Mushanga op. cit.

Rouse, J. (1985) 'Deinstitutionalization and its Impact on Swedish Corrections'. *International Journal of Comparative and Applied Criminal Justice*. 9, 71–83.

Sagarin, E. (ed.) (1980) *Taboos in Criminology*. Beverly Hills, CA: Sage.

Sahay, G. (1981) 'Probation in India'. *Indian Journal of Criminology and Criminalistics*. 1, 50–54.

Saiger, L. (1992) 'Probation Management Structures and Partnerships in America: Lessons for England'. In R. Statham and P. Whitehead op. cit.

Schermerhorn, R. (1970) *Comparative Ethnic Relations: a Framework for Theory and Research*. New York: Random House.

Scheuch, E. (1990) 'The Development of Comparative Research: Towards Causal Explanations'. In E. Øyen op. cit.

Shah, J. (1974) 'Probation Services in India'. *International Journal of Offender Therapy and Comparative Criminology*. 18, 187–191.

Shaw, R. and Haines, K. (eds) *The Criminal Justice System: a Central Role for the Probation Service*. Cambridge: University of Cambridge Institute of Criminology.

Silverman, M. (1993) 'Ethical Issues in the Field of Probation'. *International Journal of Offender Therapy and Comparative Criminology*. 37, 85–94.

Singh, D. (1980) 'Probation and Confession'. *Social Defence*. 16, 33–39.

Singh, M. (1987) *Crime and Redemption of Criminals: Probation of Offenders*. New Delhi: Deep and Deep.

Sluder, R., Shearer, R. and Potts, D. (1991) 'Probation Officers' Role Perceptions and Attitudes Toward Firearms'. *Federal Probation*. LV, 3–11.

Snyder, F. (1982) 'Colonialism and Legal Form: the Creation of "Customary Law" in Senegal'. In C. Sumner op. cit.

Spiess, G. and Johnson, E. (1980) 'Role Conflict and Role Ambiguity in Probation: Structural Sources and Consequences in West Germany. *International Journal of Comparative and Applied Criminal Justice*. 4, 179–189.

Spitzer, S. and Simon, R. (eds) (1982) *Research in Law, Deviance and Social Control: a Research Annual*. Volume 4. Greenwich, CT: JAI Press Inc.

Srivastava, S. (1987) *The Probation System: an Evaluative Study*. Lucknow: Print House.

Statham, R. and Whitehead, P. (eds) (1992) *Managing the Probation Service: Issues for the 1990s*. Harlow: Longman.

Stewart, V. (1982) *Justice and Troubled Children Around the World*. New York: New York University Press.

Sumner, C. (ed.) (1982) *Crime, Justice and Underdevelopment*. London: Heinemann.

Tadanir, N. (1969) 'Probation in Israel: Social Background and Practical Problems'. *International Journal of Offender Therapy*. 13, 111–116.

Tandon, S. (1988) 'Probationers View the Probation System'. *Indian Journal of Criminology*. 16, 47–52.

Taylor, I., Walton, P. and Young, J. (1973) *The New Criminology: for a Social Theory of Deviance*. London: Routledge and Kegan Paul.

Terrill, R. (1992) *World Criminal Justice Systems*. Cincinatti, OH: Anderson.

Thomas, J. (1972) *The English Prison Officer Since 1850: a Study in Conflict*. London: Routledge and Kegan Paul.

Tohichem, L. (1991) *Papua New Guinea Probation Service: Annual Report for 1990 to Minister for Justice and Attorney-General Honourable Bernard Narokobi LLB, MP*. Port Moresby: Acting Government Printer.

Trought, T. (1927) *Probation in Europe*. Oxford: Basil Blackwell.

United Nations (1951) *Probation and Related Measures*. Document E/CN.5/230. New York: United Nations.

United Nations (1954a) *European Seminar on Probation. London 20–30 October 1952*. Document ST/TAA/SER.C/11. New York: United Nations.

United Nations (1954b) *Practical Results and Financial Aspects of Adult Probation in Selected Countries*. Document S/SOA/SD/3. New York: United Nations.

United Nations (1959) *The Selection of Offenders for Probation*. Document ST/SOA/SD/7. New York: United Nations.

United Nations (1990) *Eighth United Nations Congress on the Prevention of Crime and the Treatment of Offenders*. Document A/Conf 144/28/Rev 1, 1990. New York: United Nations.

UNAFEI (United Nations Asia and Far East Institute for the Prevention of Crime and the Treatment of Offenders) (1980) *Alternatives to Imprisonment in Asia*. Tokyo: UNAFEI.

United Nations Interregional Crime and Justice Research Institute (1993) *International Survey on Probation Systems and Services: International Bibliography*. Rome: UNICRI.

United Nations Social Defence Research Institute (1976) *Juvenile Justice: an International Survey*. Publication No. 12. Rome: UNSDRI.

Vagg, J. (1993) 'Context and Linkage: Reflections on Comparative Research and "Internationalism' in Criminology" '. *British Journal of Criminology*. 33, 541–554.

van Swaaningen, R. and uit Beijerse, J. (1993) 'From Punishment to Diversion and Back Again: the Debate on Non-Custodial Sanctions and Penal Reform in the Netherlands'. *Howard Journal of Criminal Justice.* 32, 136–156.

Versele, S. (1969) 'Probation in Belgium'. *International Journal of Offender Therapy.* 13, 100–106.

Walczak, S. (1969) 'Probation in Poland'. *International Journal of Offender Therapy.* 13, 117–119.

Walczak, S. (1976) 'The Evolution of Probation Measures in Poland: Conditional Supervision of Criminal Proceedings'. *International Journal of Offender Therapy and Comparative Criminology.* 20, 71–72.

Walker, E. (1989) 'The Community Intensive Treatment for Youth Program: a Specialized Community-Based Program for High Risk Youth in Alabama'. *Law and Psychology Review.* 13, 175–199.

Walker, N. (1985) *Sentencing: Theory, Law and Practice.* London: Butterworth.

Webb, P. (1982) *A History of Custodial and Related Penalties in New Zealand.* Wellington: New Zealand Government Printer.

Webb, S. and Webb, B. (1922) *English Prisons Under Local Government.* London: Longmans, Green and Co.

Wegener, H. (1991) 'The Development of Non-Custodial Social Services in the Justice Setting in the New Federal States'. *Bewärungshilfe.* 38. Summarized in *Criminology, Penology and Police Science Abstracts* (1992) 32(6), 85.

Wheeler, G., Macan, T., Hissong, R. and Slusher, M. (1989) 'The Effects of Probation Service Fees on Case Management Strategies and Sanctions'. *Journal of Criminal Justice.* 17, 15–24.

Whitehead, T. (1989) *Burnout in Probation and Corrections.* New York: Praeger.

Whitehead, T. and Lindquist, C. (1992) 'Determinants of Probation and Parole Officer Professional Orientation'. *Journal of Criminal Justice.* 20, 13–24.

Wills, D. (1981) *Crime and Punishment in Revolutionary Paris.* Westport, CT: Greenwood Press.

Wilson, J. and Herrnstein, R. (1985) *Crime and Human Nature: the Definitive Study of the Causes of Crime.* New York: Simon and Schuster.

Wilson, K. and James, A. (eds) (1995) *Child Abuse: a Reader for Practitioners.* London: Baillière Tindall.

Woelinga, D. (1990) 'Probation Service and Public Opinion in the Netherlands'. *Howard Journal of Criminal Justice.* 29, 246–260.

Zvekic, U. (ed.) (1994) *Alternatives to Imprisonment in Comparative Perspective.* Chicago: Nelson-Hall.

Zvekic, U. and Alvazzi del Frate, A. (1994) *Alternatives to Imprisonment in Comparative Perspective: Bibliography.* Chicago: Nelson-Hall.

Name index

Abadinsky, H. 20
Abrahamse, A. 7
Allen, G. 20
Allen, H. 20
Alvazzi del Frate, A. 20
Ancel, M. 42, 43, 44, 45, 46, 64
Armer, M. 14, 17
Armstrong, T. 34
Augustus, John 28
Ayscough, H. 28

Bartollas, C. 20
Beijerse, J. uit 49
Bell, M. 28, 29, 64
Besinger, G. 20
Berting, J. 13
Bhattacharyya, S. 20, 37, 38
Bien, T. 193
Bishop, N. 20
Blomberg, T. 34
Blos, P. 9
Bochel, D. 21, 32
Braithwaite, J. 89, 194
Breda, R. 20
Brillon, Y. xiii
Brockman, J. 20
Brown, P. 30
Brownlee, I. 34
Brydensholt, H. 20
Bynum, T. 6
Byrne, J. 30, 34

Carpenter, M. 59
Cartledge, C. 4, 11, 20, 42, 47, 54, 101

Chakrabarti, N. 20, 38, 39
Chute, C. 28, 29, 64
Clear, T. xiii, 11, 12, 20, 21
Clifford, W. xiii, 20
Cohen, B.-Z. 20
Cohen, S. xiii, 6, 51, 194
Cole, G. 20
Cook 29
Croft, J. 12

Davies, M. 10
Diana, L. 28
Doleschal 12
Donzelot, J. 7
Downes, D. 50
Dressler, D. 29
Durst, D. 19

Edholm, L. 20
Egglestone, E. 71
Ekstedt, J. 40
Elder, J. 18
Eskridge, C. 20, 39

Fabiano, E.A. 166
Falkowski-Tucker, T. 20, 27
Farrell, M. 20
Farrington, D. 20
Faulkner, D. 62
Ferracuti, F. 20
Fielder, M. 21
Fielding, N. 26
Findlay, M. 15, 20
Fink, A. 61–2

Subject index